The Journal of the International Society for
Oncodevelopmental Biology and Medicine (ISOBM)

TumorBiology

Tumor Markers, Tumor Targeting and Translational Cancer Research

Founded 1980 as 'Oncodevelopmental Biology and Medicine' by the ISOBM, continued 1984–1986 as 'Tumour Biology'.
Former Editors: W.H. Fishman 1980–1983, H. Hirai 1980–1993, A.M. Neville 1984–1994, S. von Kleist 1995–1999.

KARGER

Printed in Switzerland
on acid-free paper by
Reinhardt Druck, Basel

Appears bimonthly:
1 volume per year
(6 issues)

Guidelines for Authors

TumorBiology

Aims and Scope

Tumor Biology is an international journal publishing original research and reviews in experimental and clinical cancer research. Translational research with a focus on tumor markers and tumor targeting are major interests of the journal, but studies in other areas of basic or clinical cancer research are also welcome.

Submission

Original manuscripts written in English should be sent to the Managing Editor:

Dr. Phil. D. Rye
Central Laboratory
The Norwegian Radium Hospital Montebello
N–0310 Oslo (Norway)
Fax +47 22 73 07 25
E-mail phil.rye@labmed.uio.no

Manuscripts should be submitted in quadruplicate with four sets of original illustrations. A disk version with manuscript and illustrations should be sent *only* after the editor's final decision for acceptance has been given. For details refer to 'Disk Submission' or www.karger.com/journals/disksub.htm. **The final version of the manuscript should match the file on disk exactly.** Editorial and copyediting will be executed from the disk version of your manuscript.

Reviews: Review articles are usually by invitation only. However, proposals clearly outlining a theme including a probable submission date are welcome. Suggestions for articles can be submitted by e-mail to the Editor-in-Chief:

Prof. Torgny Stigbrand
Department of Immunology
torgny.stigbrand@climi.umu.se

Conditions

All manuscripts are subject to peer review. Manuscripts are received with the explicit understanding that they are not under simultaneous consideration by any other publication. A cover letter with the name, address, telephone and fax numbers of the corresponding author must accompany each manuscript. This letter must include a statement that affirms that all authors agree with the submission. Submission of an article for publication implies the transfer of the copyright from the author to the publisher upon acceptance. Accepted papers become the permanent property of *Tumor Biology* and may not be reproduced by any means, in whole or in part, without the written consent of the publisher and the Editor-in-Chief. It is the author's responsibility to obtain permission to reproduce illustrations, tables, etc. from other publications.

Arrangement

The complete manuscript (including table legends, figure legends and references) should be typed double-spaced using a 12 point font on one side of the paper (A4 size or 8½ × 11 inches) with 2.5 cm (1 inch) margins on all sides and with page numbers. Articles should contain: title page, Key Words, Abstract, Introduction, Materials and Methods, Results, Discussion, Acknowledgements, References, Tables and figure legends.

Title page: The first page of each paper should indicate the title, the authors' names, and the institute where the work was done, a short title for use as running header, and the full postal address (including phone, fax and e-mail) of the corresponding author.

Key words: For indexing purposes, a list of 3–10 key words in English is essential.

Abstract: Each paper requires an abstract of up to 200 words clearly outlining the objective(s), methods, results, and conclusion(s).

Footnotes: Avoid footnotes. When essential, number consecutively and type at the foot of the appropriate page.

Tables and illustrations: Tables and illustrations (both numbered in Arabic numerals) should be prepared on separate sheets. Tables require a heading and figures a legend, also prepared on a separate sheet. For the reproduction of illustrations, only good drawings and original photographs can be accepted; negatives or photocopies cannot be used. Due to technical reasons, figures with a screen background should not be submitted. When possible, group several illustrations on one block for reproduction (max. size 181×223 mm) or provide crop marks. On the back of each illustration, indicate its number, the author's name, and 'top' with a soft pencil.

Color illustrations: Up to 6 color illustrations per page can be integrated within the text at the reduced price of CHF 660.–/USD 545.00 per page. Color illustrations are reproduced at the author's expense.

References: In the text identify references by Arabic numerals [in square brackets]. The number of references should not normally exceed 30. Material submitted for publication but not yet accepted should be noted as 'unpublished data' and not included in the reference list. The list of references should include only those publications which are cited in the text. Do not alphabetize; number references in the order in which they are first mentioned in the text. The surnames of the authors followed by initials should be given. There should be no punctuation other than a comma to separate the authors. Cite all authors, 'et al.' is not sufficient. Abbreviate journal names according to the Index Medicus system. (Also see International Committee of Medical Journal Editors: Uniform requirements for manuscripts submitted to biomedical journals. N Engl J Med 1997;336: 309–315.)

Examples

(a) Papers published in periodicals: Sun J, Koto H, Chung KF: Interaction of ozone and allergen challenges on bronchial responsiveness and inflammation in sensitised guinea pigs. Int Arch Allergy Immunol 1997;112:191–195.

(b) Monographs: Matthews DE, Farewell VT: Using and Understanding Medical Statistics, ed 3, revised. Basel, Karger, 1996.

(c) Edited books: Parren PWIII, Burton DR: Antibodies against HIV-1 from phage display libraries: Mapping of an immune response and progress towards antiviral immunotherapy; in Capra JD (ed): Antibody Engineering. Chem Immunol. Basel, Karger, 1997, vol 65, pp 18–56.

(d) Papers published in electronic format: Black CA: Delayed type hypersensitivity: Current theories with a historic perspective. Dermatol Online J 1999;5:7.
http://dermatology.cdlib.org/DOJvol5 num1.

Page Charges

There are no page charges for Research Articles of 4 (ISOBM members and subscribers: 6) or fewer printed pages (including tables, illustrations and references). Each additional complete or partial page is charged to the author at CHF 240.– / USD 150.00. One printed page is equal to approximately 3 manuscript pages (including tables, illustrations and references).

Galley proofs

Unless indicated otherwise, galley proofs are sent to the first-named author and should be returned with the least possible delay. Alterations made in galley proofs, other than the correction of printer's errors, are charged to the author. No page proofs are supplied.

Reprints

Order forms and a price list are sent with the galley proofs. Orders submitted after the issue is printed are subject to considerably higher prices.

KARGER

Fax + 41 61 306 12 34
E-Mail karger@karger.ch
www.karger.com

The Guidelines for Authors are available at:
www.karger.com/journals/tbi/tbi_gl.htm

General Information

Tumor Biology

Publication data: 'Tumor Biology' is published 6 times a year. Volume 23 with 6 issues appears in 2002.

Subscription rates: Subscriptions run for a full calendar year. Prices are given per volume.

Personal subscription:
Subscription + postage and handling
CHF 472.– + CHF 28.80 Europe
CHF 472.– + CHF 42.70 Overseas
USD 363.00 + USD 28.80
+ online subscription per volume:
CHF 39.– / USD 30.00
(Must be in the name of, billed to, and paid by an individual. Order must be marked 'personal subscription'.)

Institutional subscription:
Subscription + postage and handling
CHF 944.– + CHF 36.– Europe
CHF 944.– + CHF 53.40 Overseas
USD 726.00 + USD 36.00
+ online subscription per volume:
CHF 58.– / USD 45.00

Airmail postage: CHF 36.–, USD 30.00. (Extra per volume.)

Discount subscription prices: American Association for Cancer Research; European Association for Cancer Research; Japanese Cancer Association. Tumor Biology is included in 'International Society for Oncodevelopmental Biology and Medicine (ISOBM)' membership fee, for information: http://www.med.uio.no/isobm

Microforms: Please direct all enquiries and orders to:
University Microfilms Inc.
300 North Zeeb Road, P.O. Box 1346
Ann Arbor, MI 48106-1346 (USA)

Subscription orders: Orders can be placed at agencies, bookstores, directly with the
Publisher S. Karger AG, P.O. Box,
CH–4009 Basel (Switzerland)
or with any of the following distributors:
Deutschland: S. Karger GmbH, Postfach
D–79095 Freiburg
France: Librairie Luginbühl
36, bd de Latour-Maubourg
F–75007 Paris
Great Britain, Ireland: S. Karger AG
4 Rickett Street
London SW6 1RU, UK
USA: S. Karger Publishers, Inc.
26 West Avon Road, P.O. Box 529
Farmington, CT 06085, USA
India, Bangladesh, Sri Lanka:
Panther Publishers Private Ltd.
33, First Main
Koramangala First Block
Bangalore 560 034, India
Japan: Karger Japan, Inc.
Yushima S Bld. 3F
4-2-3, Yushima, Bunkyo-ku
Tokyo 113-0034, Japan

Change of address: Both old and new address should be sent to the subscription source.

Advertising: Correspondence and rate requests should be addressed to the Publisher.

Single issues and back volumes: Information can be obtained through the Publisher.

Bibliographic indices: This journal is regularly listed in bibliographic services, including *Current Contents®*.

Book Reviews: Books are accepted for review by special agreement.

Copying: This journal has been registered with the Copyright Clearance Center (CCC), as indicated by the code appearing on the first page of each article.
For readers in the US, this code signals consent for copying of articles for personal or internal use, or for the personal or internal use of specific clients, provided that the stated fee is paid per copy directly to
Copyright Clearance Center Inc.
222 Rosewood Drive
Danvers, MA 01923 (USA).
A copy of the first page of the article must accompany payment. Consent does not extend to copying for general distribution, for promotion, for creating new works, or for resale. In these cases, specific written permission must be obtained from the copyright owner,
S. Karger AG, P.O. Box,
CH–4009 Basel (Switzerland).

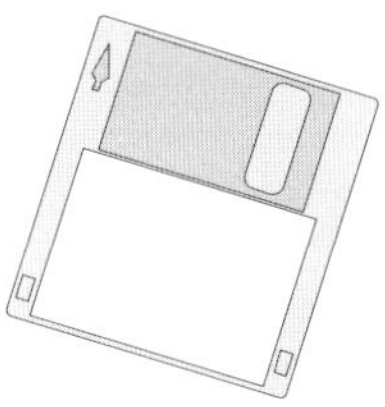

Disk Submission

A **comprehensive version** of these guidelines for the **submission of manuscripts and illustrations on disk** can be accessed online under **www.karger.com/journals/disksub.htm** or requested as a leaflet from the editorial department.

Please follow the general rules on style and arrangement in the **'Guidelines for Authors'** of the journal. Submit a **double-spaced printout** of your manuscript matching the file on disk exactly.

Technical Information

Store only data pertinent to this manuscript. Include your fonts (screen and printer fonts for Macintosh).
For a **text only** manuscript, use a 3.5-inch disk. For **text and illustrations,** use 3.5 or 5.25 Magneto Optical Disc; CD-ROM (DOS or hybrid); iomage Zip/DOS (100 MB), or 44 MB, 88 MB or 200 MB SyQuest. Compress extensive data using ZIP format.

Data Description

Label your disk with the **title of the journal or book** for which it is submitted; a **short version** of the paper's title; your **name,** postal and e-mail address, fax and phone number; **hard- and software** used, including the version; and the **complete list of the file names.** File names consist of eight characters before the dot identifying the file and three characters after the dot identifying the application.

Text and Format

The **preferred word-processing package is MS-Word.** Other commonly used PC text programs and ASCII formats are accepted.
Update your data when you revise subsequent to the reviewer's or editor's decision and mark revisions clearly. Manuscripts accepted for publication are subject to **copy editing:** changes and/or questions will be marked in the manuscript, which will be returned to you with your disk and the galley proofs for checking.
Enter your text continuously flush left. Do not use any layout functions. Do not split words at the end of a line. **Do not use indentations.** Use a blank line before and a hard return at the end of paragraphs. **Arrange headings flush left.** Insert only **one space after punctuation marks.** Insert Greek letters, mathematical symbols etc. with your word-processing program. Use **boldface and italics** as well as sub- and superscript where appropriate. **Tables are part of the text** and should be placed at the end of the text file. Separate the individual parts of a table by lines. Use the tabulator instead of spaces. Format operation data on one line in the same column. **Legends to illustrations are part of the text** and should also be listed at the end of the text file.

Illustrations

Store illustrations as separate files: do not integrate them in your text. Export **line drawings/vector graphics** as TIF, EPS or WMF format. Use Photoshop for processing and retouching **scanned half-tone images.** Save the original scan and the processed version. Export **black and white or color images** as TIF or EPS format in their anticipated size in print.
For detailed information on how to submit illustration data on disk please consult the leaflet or **www.karger.com/journals/disksub.htm.**

KARGER

Fax +41 61 306 12 34
E-Mail karger@karger.ch
www.karger.com

The Journal Home Page is available at:
www.karger.com/journals/tbi

KI 98 DISK

TumorBiology

Translational Cancer Research

Abstracts

The XXXth Meeting of the International Society for Oncodevelopmental Biology and Medicine, ISOBM 2002, September 8–12, 2002, Boston, Mass.

Organizer
Herbert Z. Kupchik, Boston, Mass.

KARGER

Basel · Freiburg · Paris · London · New York ·
New Delhi · Bangkok · Singapore · Tokyo · Sydney

S. Karger
Medical and Scientific Publishers
Basel · Freiburg · Paris · London
New York · New Delhi · Bangkok
Singapore · Tokyo · Sydney

Drug Dosage
The authors and the publisher have exerted every effort to ensure that drug selection and dosage set forth in this text are in accord with current recommendations and practice at the time of publication. However, in view of ongoing research, changes in government regulations, and the constant flow of information relating to drug therapy and drug reactions, the reader is urged to check the package insert for each drug for any change in indications and dosage and for added warnings and precautions. This is particularly important when the recommended agent is a new and/or infrequently employed drug.

P.O. Box, CH–4009 Basel (Switzerland)
Printed in USA by RP Graphics, Pinehurst, Mass.
ISBN 3–8055–7478–9

KARGER

Fax + 41 61 306 12 34
E-Mail karger@karger.ch
www.karger.com

S-1

SIGNAL TRANSDUCTION BY JNK

Roger J. Davis
Howard Hughes Medical Institute and University of Massachusetts Medical School, Worcester, MA

The JNK group of stress-activated MAP kinases consists of ten protein kinases that phosphorylate the NH_2-terminal activation domain of c-Jun on Ser-63 and Ser-73 causing increased transcriptional activity (1, 2). JNK protein kinase activity is increased in response to treatment of cells with pro-inflammatory cytokines or exposure to environmental stress. Activated JNK is phosphorylated on Thr and Tyr within the tripeptide motif Thr-Pro-Tyr located in kinase sub-domain VIII. Mutational analysis demonstrates that JNK activation requires the phosphorylation of both Thr and Tyr within this motif. This phosphorylation is mediated by dual specificity protein kinases, including MKK4 and MKK7 (3). This phosphorylation can be potentiated, under some physiological conditions, by the interaction of these protein kinases with members of the JIP group of scaffold proteins (4).

The function of the JNK signaling pathway has been studied using a combination of biochemical and genetic approaches. Genetic analysis of JNK signaling in *Drosophila* demonstrates that JNK is required for early embryonic morphogenesis. Similarly, disruption of the JNK signaling pathway in mice using homologous recombination demonstrates that JNK is required for embryonic viability (1,2). The defects include changes in stress-induced gene expression and apoptosis (4). These studies provide insight into the role of the JNK stress-activated MAP kinase pathway in the cellular response to environmental stress, including radiation. The role of JNK in tumor development will be discussed.

References

1. Davis, R. J. “Signal transduction by the JNK group of MAP kinases” Cell 103, 239-252 (2000).
2. Weston, C. R. and Davis, R. J. “The JNK signal transduction pathway” Curr. Opin. Genet. Dev. 12, 14-21 (2002).
3. Tournier, C., Dong, C., Turner, T. K., Jones, S. N., Flavell, R. A., and Davis, R. J. “MKK7 is an essential component of the JNK signal transduction pathway activated by pro-inflammatory cytokines” Genes & Dev. 15, 1419-1426 (2001).
4. Whitmarsh, A. J., Kuan, C-Y., Kennedy, N. J., Kelkar, N., Haydar, T., Mordes, J. P., Appel, M., Rossini, A. A., Jones, S. N., Flavell,R. A., Rakic, P., and Davis, R. J. “Requirement of the JIP1 scaffold protein for stress-induced JNK activation” Genes & Dev. 15, 2421-2432 (2001).
5. Tournier, C., Hess, P., Yang, D. D., Xu, J., Turner, T. K., Nimnual, A., Bar-Sagi, D., Jones, S. N., Flavell, R. A., and Davis, R. J.
“Requirement of JNK for stress-induced activation of the cytochrome c-mediated death pathway” Science 288, 870-874 (2000).

S-2

CLINICAL APPLICATION OF MOLECULAR TARGETS

Ed Sausville
National Cancer Institute, Bethesda, MD

The paradigm for cancer drug discovery and development has in the last decade undergone a profound change. Prior to 1990, cancer drugs for the most part manifested initial evidence of anti-proliferative activity in tumor cells growing either *in vitro* or *in vivo* in animals. Empirical anti-tumor activity was optimized in tumor models usually selected without reference to the compound's mechanism of action. Initial Phase I trials defined a maximum tolerated dose on a particular schedule, and this schedule was advanced to Phase II studies seeking to define tumor shrinkage as a surrogate for useful activity that favorably influenced the survival of treated patients. While a substantial fraction of the currently available anti-cancer drugs were discovered and developed in this way, this process was inefficient and did not take into account the biology of the tumor. The explosion of information relating to the biology of cancer has raised the hypothesis that targeting specific molecules or processes important in the pathogenesis of cancer will lead to useful therapeutic agents. Ideally, drug discovery activities, up to and including early phase clinical trials would incorporate biologic information into the plan for a drug's development. Early examples of this shift of thinking include the relative success of Herceptin® and Gleevec®, targeting HER2/NEU and BCR/ABL or KIT, respectively. However, numerous questions remain in applying this model in the hopes of more broad success. These include how to validate targets as suitable for therapeutic intervention? When and how to use assays of drug effect in surrogate or tumor tissue from patients? How to choose combinations of agents affecting different pathways? Should dose escalation proceed to toxicity or to the demonstration of a biologically effective dose? Examples illustrating potential approaches to the issues will be provided, and an approach that recognizes four classes of molecular targets relevant to clinical development outlined: *Pathogenic* targets relate to the molecular events related to a tumor's neoplastic transformation; *ontogenic* targets relate to the tissue or cell type of origin; *pharmacologic* targets relate to differential drug handling by the tumor or the host; and *microenvironmental* targets reside in the anatomical interface of the tumor with the host. Each of these different types of molecular targets offer distinct challenges and opportunities, but capitalizing on their defined or definable biology in relation to drug action promises the common feature of greatly increased efficiency and intellectual rigor with which drug discovery and development schemes can be proposed and undertaken.

S-3

CHEMOPREVENTION OF HUMAN CANCERS: TARGETS, THERAPIES, AND TIMING

Marianne N. Prout, MD
Boston University School of Public Health
Boston, MA

As oncodevelopmental biology elucidates the molecular and genetic processes of carcinogenesis, translational research uses these processes as therapeutic targets for agents that may inhibit or reverse carcinogenesis. The translation of biologic models to clinical trials of chemoprevention raises issues about targets, therapies, and timing

Definitive chemoprevention trials require that biologic targets be identified in large populations. Inherited genetic markers require expensive testing that follows time-consuming, detailed knowledge of medical histories of extended families. Exposure histories may be used to select individuals to test for biologic changes, such as measurement of DNA adducts in persons exposed to aflatoxins or DNA repair capacity in smokers. Intraepithelial neoplasias and earlier precursor lesions to cancers are often identified through cancer screening of populations, e.g. colon polyps, atypical ductal hyperplasia in the breast, oral leukoplakias, atypical squamous cells of the cervix, prostatic intraepithelial neoplasia (PIN). These markers may be used as Surrogate Endpoint Biomarkers (SEB) for preliminary trials of new therapies, but chemoprevention agents must ultimately be proven effective at prevention of cancers. Thus the transformation rate and the transition time from the SEB to invasive cancer must either be known or evaluated in trials. Persons cured of cancer are a readily identified group at high risk for additional cancers. Multiple primaries occur for many common epithelial cancers associated with field cancerization, implying that individuals may have cells in multiple phases of carcinogenesis simultaneously.

Potential therapeutic agents for chemoprevention come from many broad categories: antimutagens, antiproliferative agents, antioxidants, antiinflammatoy agents, and hormonally active agents. Biologically targeted therapies, such as the Selective Estrogen Receptor Modulator tamoxifen, challenge the clear distinction between therapies for clinical cancers and therapies for precursor lesions. “Broad spectrum” or combination chemoprevention strategies are based on the probability that an individual at increased risk for cancer has cells in many phases of carcinogenesis.

The timing of chemoprevention is based on biologic data and considerations of toxicities, costs, adherence, and comorbidites, among other issues. Chemopreventive agents which address biologic processes late in carcinogenesis may be delivered in the 5-10 years preceding the rise in incidence in the population-based data. Chemopreventive agents which are targeted to biologic processes which precede cancers by 10-20 years, however, would need to be virtually free of toxicity, very low in cost, and require only short-term administration. For example tamoxifen, a suspected teratogen, is inappropriate for women who wish to bear children. Cyclooxygenase-2 inhibitors may have a better therapeutic ratio than aspirin for chemoprevention of colon cancers.

S-4

TUMOR MARKER ASSAYS: THEIR ROLE AND RELEVANCE

Morton K. Schwartz
Memorial Sloan Kettering Cancer Center, New York, NY

Although biochemical makers have been used in the management of cancer patients for more than a century, it was not until the introduction of isotopic assay procedures that the term tumor marker came into use and was applied to measurement of tumor related proteins in serum. This definition has been enlarged to include tissue materials, receptors and most recently oncogenes and their products. There are now more than a dozen FDA approved tumor markers and many more than that are used world-wide, but not approved for routine use in the United States. The major controversy is their use in medical practice as whether this can improve survival, reduce morbidity and improve the quality of life of the cancer patient and their role and their relevance in the management of the cancer patient. What is the responsibility of the laboratory, the laboratory scientist and the clinician in defining this role. Carcinoembryonic antigen (CEA) is the oldest of the "new" markers. It is in our clinical laboratory the often requested tumor marker tests. We now know a great deal about the genetics and biochemistry of the molecule but its clinical role and use is still misunderstood. Its role in prognosis will be reviewed as well as its use in monitoring with the realization that "second look surgery" based on CEA apparently does not improve survival but may improve quality of life. Alpha-feto protein (AFP) and Beta-human chorionic gonadotropin (b-hCG) in germ cell tumors are the unique example of a marker combination which combined with specific therapy results in "cures" in a previously incurable and fatal disease. These markers lead us into discussions of the role of algorithms with tumor markers and the need for absolute standardization. Prostate specific antigen (PSA) is described as a specific organ related marker. It has been widely accepted a a marker to assist in diagnosis and to monitor therapy. Despite controversy it is now FDA approved for use in "screening". Unfortunately it in itself cannot differentiate aggressive from non aggressive tumors. Extensive laboratory work and clinical studies are underway to improve the absolute sensitivity and specificity of PSA. Breast Cancer patient management has been supplemented for many years by tumor receptor assays and monitoring in serum of patients of glycoprotein markers such as CA15-3. These markers are only elevated in the presence of extensive disease but cannot predict response or exacerbation of disease. Recently Herceptin, a monoclonal antibody directed against the HER 2/neu receptor has been successful in treating women with metastatic breast cancer who express HER 2/neu in their tissue. The assay of HER2/neu can be a predictive marker of therapy and prognosis. A serum assay of HER2/neu has demonstrated similar findings to the tissue assays, but also permits sequential monitoring and allows evaluation of therapy over time. All of the tumor markers have assisted in the positive results in cancer care, but the serious problem remains of the difference in values by the many methods in use, the quality of standardization and the required precision of the assays. What is needed is a clear understanding of each tumor marker by both the uses and the provider concerning the capabilities of the test, the biological role of the marker and whether combinations of markers are more useful than single use.

S-5

THE DIAGNOSTIC UTILITY OF GROWTH FACTOR RECEPTORS AND THEIR CIRCULATING FRAGMENTS

Walter P. Carney, PhD
Oncogene Science/Bayer Diagnostics, Cambridge, MA

Growth Factor Receptors such as Epidermal Growth Factor Receptor (EGFR, also called HER-1), Human Epidermal Growth Factor Receptor-2 (HER-2) are located on the surface of epithelial cells and when stimulated by various ligands initiate a cascade of intracellular signals resulting in cell proliferation. For many years, scientists have been investigating the role of these and other growth factor receptors (FLT-1, KDR) in the initiation and progression of various cancers. HER-2/neu and EGFR are part of a larger family of growth factor receptors, which include HER-3 and HER-4. HER-1 through HER-4 are members of a family of human erbB genes that are structurally and functionally related to the viral erbB (v-erbB) oncogene carried by a retrovirus.

It was shown more than 50 years ago that retroviral oncogenes encode oncoproteins that contribute to converting normal cells to cancer cells. In the early 1980's, several groups showed that HER-2/neu and EGFR DNA sequences found in human cancer cells were structurally similar to the v-erbB retroviral oncogene. Subsequent studies showed that DNA from either HER-2/neu and EGFR could convert normal cells to cells with malignant properties and have been referred to as Oncogenes. For more than 10 years, there 2 growth factor receptors/oncogenes have been extensively studied and are targets for the development of a new class of cancer therapeutics.

EGFR and HER-2/neu are both transmembrane tyrosine kinase receptors that are overexpressed in some cancer cells. The full-length HER-2/neu oncoprotein has a molecular weight of 185,000 daltons whereas the EGFR has a molecular weight of 170,000 daltons. Both proteins are composed of 3 parts, an internal tyrosine kinase portion, responsible for intracellular signaling, a short transmembrane portion and the extracellular domain (ECD) which is the portion that interacts with various ligands. The ECDs of both EGFR and HER-2/neu have been shown to be released from the cell surface and have been found to circulate in normal people and cancer patients. The shed ECD of HER-2/neu is a glycoprotein between 97,000 and 115,00 daltons and has been referred to as p105 whereas the ECD for EGFR is 110,000 daltons and referred to as p110. The shed ECDs from either HER-2/neu and EGFR can be measured in serum or plasma using antibody based immunoassays.

In contrast to tissue testing, serum/plasma testing allows a real time assessment of a patient's HER-2/neu and EGFR status, allows repeat testing for patient monitoring and can be performed in a standardized and quantitative manner. This presentation will focus the clinical utility of measuring the circulating ECDs of HER-2/neu and EGFR in several epithelial cancers and will discuss the potential role of these assays in both monitoring patients receiving HER-2/neu and EGFR directed therapies.

S-6

ANGIOGENESIS AND LYMPHANGIOGENESIS IN TUMORS: NEW INSIGHTS FROM INTRAVITAL MICROSCOPY

Rakesh K. Jain
Radiation Oncology, Massachusetts General Hospital, Harvard Medical School, Boston, MA

The past 30 years have witnessed unprecedented advances in our understanding of the molecular origins of cancer and other diseases. These advances have led to the identification of numerous genes associated with oncogenesis and the development of a wide variety of novel therapeutics. The grand challenge now is (i) to relate expression of these genes with their function *in vivo*, and (ii) to deliver these novel therapeutics to their targets *in vivo* in optimal quantities. Most methods used today to address these questions are either invasive or have poor spatial resolution. To overcome these problems we developed a number of transparent windows in animals (1). We also developed transgenic cell lines and mice that express GFP when the gene of interest is switched on (2). Using intravital microscopy and computer-assisted image analysis we can visualize and quantify gene expression, physiological function and micro-pharmacokinetics (3). This approach has allowed us to gain powerful insight into angiogenesis as well as the physiological barriers to the delivery and effectiveness of therapeutic agents in tumors (4,5). In my presentation today, I will discuss our recent findings on the critical role of host-tumor interaction in tumor growth, angiogenesis, lymphangiogenesis and response to therapies. I will demonstrate that cancer cells co-opt the host cells into producing pro- and anti- angiogenic molecules (6,7) as well as the extracellular matrix molecules (8). Since host cells are different in each organ, the biology of tumors is host-organ dependant. These findings may explain why successful responses to various therapies seen in subcutaneous tumors in mice do not always predict the response in patients where the tumors arise in other organs. I will present a counter-intuitive strategy to overcome the physiological barriers by anti-angiogenic approaches (7,9). Finally, I will present our recent data on function of lymphatic vessels in transplanted and spontaneous tumors (10, 11).

1. R.K. Jain, L.L. Munn and D. Fukumura, "Dissecting Tumour Pathophysiology Using Intravital Microscopy," Nature Reviews Cancer, 2: 266-276 (2002).
2. D. Fukumura, R. Xavier, T. Sugiura, Y. Chen, E.C. Parks, N. Lu, M. Selig, G. Nielsen, T. Taksir, R.K. Jain and B. Seed, "Tumor Induction of VEGF Promoter Activity in Stromal Cells," Cell, 94: 715-725 (1998).
3. E.B. Brown, R.B. Campbell, Y. Tsuzuki, L. Xu, P. Carmeliet, D. Fukumura, and R.K. Jain, "In vivo measurement of gene expression, angiogenesis and physiological function in tumors using multiphoton laser scanning microscopy," Nature Medicine, 7(7): 864-8 (2001).
4. R.K. Jain, "Barriers to Drug Delivery in Solid Tumors," Scientific American, 271: 58-65 (1994).
5. R.K. Jain, "Delivery of Molecular Medicine to Solid Tumors: Lessons from In Vivo Imaging of Gene Expression and Function," J Controlled Release, 74: 7-25 (2001).
6. T. Gohongi, D. Fukumura, Y. Boucher, C. Yun, G.A. Soff, C. Compton, T. Todoroki and R.K. Jain, "Tumor-host Interactions in the Gallbladder Suppress Distal Angiogenesis and Tumor Growth: Role of TGFb," Nature Medicine, 5: 1203-1208 (1999).
7. Y. Izumi, L. Xu, E. di Tomaso, D. Fukumura, and R.K. Jain, "Herceptin Acts as an Anti-Angiogenic Cocktail," Nature, 416: 279-280 (2002).
8. A. Pluen, Y. Boucher, S. Ramanujan, T.D. McKee, T. Gohongi, E. di Tomaso, E.B. Brown, Y. Izumi, R.B. Campbell, D.A. Berk, R.K. Jain, "Role of Tumor-Host Interactions in Interstitial Diffusion of Macromolecules: Cranial vs. Subcutaneous Tumors," *PNAS*, **98**: 4628-4633 (2001).
9. R.K. Jain, "Normalizing Tumor Vasculature with Anti-Angiogenic Therapy: A New Paradigm for Combination Therapy," *Nature Medicine*, **7:** 987-989 (2001).
10. R.K. Jain, and B.T. Fenton, "Intra-Tumoral Lymphatics: A Case of Mistaken Identity or Malfunction?" *JNCI* **94:** 417-421 (2002)
11. T.P. Padera, E. di Tomaso, A. Kadambi, C. Mouta Carreira, E.B. Brown, Y. Boucher, N.C. Choi, D. Mathisen, J. Wain, E.J. Mark, L.L. Munn, R.K. Jain, "Lymphatic Metastasis in the Absence of Functional Intratumor Lymphatics," *Science*, 296:1883-1886, (2002).

S-7

MICROARRAYS AND ONCODEVELOPMENTAL BIOLOGY OF THE LUNG

Jerome S. Brody, Avrum Spira
Pulmonary Center and Department of Medicine, Boston University School of Medicine, Boston, MA

Microarrays, which provide simultaneous measures of the expression levels of thousands of genes, have been increasingly applied to understanding tumor and developmental biology in many tissues and in many species over the past several years. Gene expression profiles derived from microarrays have been used for classification, diagnosis, prognosis, and decisions about treatment as well as defining basic mechanisms of cell transformation and carcinogenesis in many tissues. They have also been used to explore basic mechanisms of organogenesis and of cellular differentiation.

To illustrate the impact of microarrays in oncodevelopmental biology, we will present recent studies from our laboratory that focus on two tobacco-related diseases; pulmonary emphysema and lung cancer. Expression profiles of lung tissue from smokers with lung cancer, emphysema, or normal lungs and correlations with airway epithelial cell gene expression will be presented. These studies have as their goals exploring differences in susceptibility to tobacco-related epithelial cell injury, defining mechanisms of early injury, developing tools for early diagnosis of disease, and defining potential targets preventative therapy. Bioinformatic techniques that relate human gene expression to yeast proteomics in order to define potential function of genes that are altered by smoke exposure will be discussed. Several examples of how microarrays can be used to explore mechanisms of lung development will be presented and expression data relating to the physiologic response to the altered lung redox state that occurs at birth will be discussed.

S-8

ANTIBODY-BASED TARGETING OF ANGIOGENESIS

Dario Neri, PhD
Institute of Pharmaceutical Sciences, Swiss Federal Institute of Technology, Zurich, Switzerland

Angiogenesis, i.e., the proliferation of new blood vessels from pre-existing ones, is an underlying process in many human diseases, including cancer, blinding ocular disorders and rheumatoid arthritis. The ability to selectively target and occlude neovasculature will be potentially useful in diagnosis and treatment of angiogenesis-related diseases.

A good-quality marker for both tumoural and non-tumoural neovasculature is the extra-domain B (ED-B) of fibronectin, a sequence of 91 aminoacids that can be inserted into the fibronectin molecule by a mechanism of alternative splicing.

To date, the production of monoclonal antibodies directly recognising the ED-B domain has not been possible using hybridoma technology, because of tolerance. In collaboration with Prof. Dr. Luciano Zardi (Istituto Nazionale per la Ricerca sul Cancro, Genova, Italy), we have overcome this problem using large synthetic antibody phage libraries, generating several high-affinity antibody fragments specific for fibronectin containing the ED-B domain, and mapping their epitope onto the three-dimensional structure of the antigen. These antibodies stain vascular structures in tumour sections and selectively target tumour neovasculature, as shown in tumour-bearing mice using infrared fluorescence and radioactive techniques. Increased binding affinity leads to improved targeting of tumoural angiogenesis, as demonstrated by biodistributions studies performed using the L19 antibody fragment with affinity for the ED-B domain in the picomolar range and L19 mutants with reduced affinity. In this lecture, I will present therapy results obtained in tumour-bearing mice treated with a number of L19-based fusion proteins. Fusion partners for the L19 antibody include tTF (a pro-coagulant factor) and anti-tumor cytokines.

The results obtained are of therapeutic relevance, since the ED-B domain of fibronectin, a naturally-occurring marker of angiogenesis identical in mouse and man, is expressed in the majority of aggressive solid tumours, but is undetectable in normal vessels and tissues.

Selected references:

B. Carnemolla, L. Borsi, E. Balza, P. Castellani, R. Meazza, A. Berndt, S. Ferrini, H. Kosmehl, D. Neri, L. Zardi. (2002) “Enhancement of the anti-tumor properties of interleukin-2 by its targeted delivery to the tumor blood vessel extracellular matrix”. *Blood*, 99, 1659-1665.

C. Halin, S. Rondini, F. Nilsson, A. Berndt, H. Kosmehl, L. Zardi, D. Neri (2002) “Enhancement of the anti-tumor activity of interleukin-12 by targeted delivery to neo-vasculature”. *Nature Biotechnol.*, 20, 264-269.

S-9

THE NEXT GENERATION OF TUMOR MARKER ASSAYS

Daniel W. Chan, PhD, DABCC, FACB
Clinical Chemistry Division, Department of Pathology, Johns Hopkins Medical Center, Baltimore, MD

With the completion of the Human Genome Project, the focus is now on functional genomics and proteomics. The next generation of tumor markers will be discovered from these new findings. Traditional tumor marker assays were developed from tumor extracts and used monoclonal antibodies. The great majority of tumor markers were used as a single marker for a particular clinical application. The next generation of assays will be based on multiple markers. It is likely that gene or protein chips will be used in combination with mass spectrometry for analysis, although monoclonal antibody based assays would probably be as cost effective for high throughput analysis. In conjunction with bioinformatics tools, this will greatly facilitate the discovery of new and better tumor markers. The high sensitivity and specificity achieved by the combined use of the selected biomarkers have great potential for the early detection of major cancers such as breast, ovarian and prostate carcinomas.

CANCER VACCINES

Jeffrey Schlom, PhD
Laboratory of Tumor Immunology and Biology, Center for Cancer Research, National Cancer Institute, National Institutes of Health, Bethesda, MD

It has now been demonstrated in both experimental models and recent clinical trials that certain "self" antigens, which are functionally non-immunogenic in the host, can become immunogenic if presented to the immune system in a certain way. Recombinant vaccines and vaccine strategies have now been developed to induce and potentiate T-cell responses of the host to such self-antigens. These strategies include: (a) The use of recombinant poxvirus vectors in which the tumor-associated antigen (TAA) is inserted as a transgene. Recombinant vaccinia vaccines and recombinant avipox (replication defective) vaccines have been employed to break tolerance to a self-antigen. (b) The use of diversified prime and boost strategies using different vaccines. (c) The insertion of T-cell costimulatory molecules into recombinant poxvirus vectors, along with the TTA gene, to enhance T-cell immune responses to the TAA. (d) The use of cytokines, such as GM-CSF and low-dose Il-2, as biological adjuvants. (e) Designing alterations in the amino acid sequence of the TAA to render it more immunogenic.

Carcinoembryonic antigen (CEA) is a self-antigen, which is expressed in fetal tissue, and overexpressed in a range of human carcinomas as compared with normal adult tissue. CEA is overexpressed in the vast majority of colorectal, pancreatic and gastric carcinomas, 70% of non-small cell lung cancers, 50% of breast cancers, and other carcinomas such as head and neck tumors. We have utilized a CEA transgenic mouse in which CEA is expressed in fetal tissue and normal tissue in a manner very similar to that of humans. While this mouse is tolerant to CEA when using CEA protein in adjuvant as a vaccine, the use of recombinant vectors expressing CEA along with the strategies outlined above have demonstrated the ability to induce strong cellular immune responses directed against CEA. Studies have also demonstrated the ability to eliminate experimental metastases expressing CEA without evidence of auto-immunity. The vaccine strategies outlined above have been translated to clinical studies in patients with advanced CEA-expressing carcinomas. These studies have demonstrated that patients can indeed mount cellular immune responses specific to CEA, which are capable of lysing CEA-expressing tumor cells. Evidence of anti-tumor activity has also been demonstrated in clinical studies.

S-11

ADHESION MOLECULES

Lucia R. Languino, Loredana Moro, Tom Manes, Mara Fornaro and Duo-Qi Zheng
Yale University, Department of Pathology, New Haven, CT

The interactions between cancer cells and extracellular matrix proteins are mediated by integrins, that have emerged as critical modulators of cell adhesion, proliferation, migration and intracellular signaling. The pathological consequences of integrin deregulated expression in cancer are the focus of current investigations. The β1 and β3 integrins are differentially expressed in normal and neoplastic cells. Our recent findings show that their expression plays a pivotal role in modulating prostate cancer cell functions *in vivo*, since they significantly affect prostate tumor growth. Using genetically engineered and primary prostate cancer cells, we have found that, *in vitro*, the β1 and β3 integrins modulate cell adhesion and motility via activation of specific signaling events and via regulation of gene expression. Studies in our laboratory aimed to identify downstream effectors of β1 and β3 integrins have unraveled two novel pathways regulated by β1 and β3 integrins that involve changes in gene expression; respectively, an IGF (insulin-like growth factor)II - mediated pathway that controls cell adhesion and a cdc2 (cyclin-dependent kinase 1, cdk1) - mediated pathway that controls cell migration. Therefore, given their deregulated expression in neoplastic cells and their ability to control multiple downstream signals, the β1 and β3 integrins and their downstream effectors provide exciting opportunities for new approaches to cancer therapy.

S-12

WHAT IS THE USE OF METASTASIS MARKERS?

Lloyd M Hutchinson, Seanna Kim, Naoko Ushiyama, Christian M Becker, Eric L Chang, Sandra M Gaston, Bruce R Zetter
Children's Hospital, Boston, MA, Beth Israel Deaconess East Campus, Boston MA, MD Anderson Cancer Center, Houston, TX

The use of genomics and proteomic techniques in recent years have identified a large number of markers associated with the metastatic state in human and animal tumors. Because the expression of these markers generally changes somewhat late in the course of tumor progression, they are not useful as simple diagnostic markers because they do not distinguish all tumors from normal tissue. Such markers may, however, be useful as prognostic or predictive markers in cancers where different treatment decisions can be made based on the progression status of a patient's cancer. For example, accurate molecular staging of prostate cancer could help distinguish between those patients that would benefit from watchful waiting versus surgery or radiological intervention. During the last 20 years, both the incidence and mortality of prostate cancer (PCa) have increased in the United States. The prostate specific antigen (PSA) test has served as an excellent diagnostic assay for the early detection of PCa, but has been of little prognostic value. Therefore, a molecular marker that can identify individuals with a tumor that is likely to metastasize, would be advantageous. Our laboratory has been working on identifying such markers. We will describe the potential role of one such marker, thymosin β15 (Tβ15) as a potential predictive marker for human prostate cancer. Tβ15 belongs to a family of highly conserved proteins which sequester monomeric actin. As such these proteins can influence the intracellular equilibrium between G- and F-actin thereby regulating cell motility, a critical component of tumor metastasis. Previously, we demonstrated that Tβ15 is expressed in metastatic PCa cells but not in nonmetastatic cells. Furthermore, Tβ15 could not be detected in normal adult tissues, a desirable quality for a tumor marker. Retrospective immunohistochemical studies have confirmed the prognostic value of Tβ15 in predicting PSA and bone failure in PCa patients. To have clinical relevance, a quantitative, high-through-put assay was needed. We have therefore developed a competition ELISA able to detect Tβ15 in urine at concentrations ranging from 10 to 1250 ng/ml. We present initial data from a prospective study evaluating tumor release of Tβ15 as a predictive indicator for metastasis and recurrent disease. Urine samples generated by an outpatient urology clinic during a one year period (>1000) including age-matched controls and other cancer types, were collected. Tβ15 ELISA values were normalized against urine concentrations of creatinine and protein to control for variability in sample concentration. Our work suggests that Tβ15 levels rare elevated at the time of PSA diagnosis in a cohort of patients, fall after treatment and rise again after PSA failure. Patients will be followed on a repeat basis to determine whether Tβ15 levels, taken at the time of diagnosis or after primary treatment, correlate with or predict PSA failure and disease recurrence.

S-13

THE "2G" INSERTION POLYMORPHISM IN THE MATRIX METALLOPROTEINASE-1 (MMP-1) PROMOTER ENHANCES INVASION IN METASTATIC MELANOMA

Constance E. Brinckerhoff, Ulrike Benbow, Colby A. Wyatt, Jonathan T. Huntington, Grant B. Tower, Walter W. Noll
Departments of Biochemistry, Medicine, Pathology, Physiology, Dartmouth Medical School
Hanover, NH

Degradation of the interstitial collagens (types I and III) in the extracellular matrix is an integral component of tumor invasion and metastasis. Much of this degradation is mediated by collagenase-1 (MMP-1), a member of the family of Matrix Metalloproteinases (MMPs). Low levels of MMP-1 expression are seen in normal physiology, but expression increases greatly in pathological conditions, such as tumor invasion and metastasis, as tumor cells and adjacent stromal cells respond to growth factors in their milieu.

We have found a single nucleotide polymorphsim (SNP) in the MMP-1 promoter that enhances transcription of this gene. Located at –1607 bp, it represents the absence or presence of an additional guanine (G), creating the sequence 5'-GAA-3' (1G allele) or 5'-GGAA-3' (2G allele). The 2G allele is a binding site for the Ets family of transcription factors, and a target of signal/transduction pathways for growth factors such as basic Fibroblast Growth Factor (bFGF). bFGF is a potent inducer of MMP-1 and is expressed by invasive melanoma cells. Therefore, we examined the influence of bFGF and the role of the 2G SNP on MMP-1 expression in malignant melanoma.

A2058 and VMM5 are two melanoma cell lines that produce high levels of MMP-1 constitutively. We investigated the mechanisms regulating this high expression. First, by RT-PCR and Western blot analysis we determined that A2058 and VMM5 melanoma cells produce bFGF, suggesting that autocrine production of bFGF drives MMP-1 expression in these cells. Growth factors often utilize the ERK1/2 signal/transduction pathway, and we used the inhibitor, PD98059, which blocks this pathway to determine whether it was controlling MMP-1 expression. In A2058 melanoma cells (2G genotype), this inhibitor (5 – 10 μM) blocked MMP-1 expression, but was only partially effective in VMM5 melanoma cells (1G genotype), suggesting that the inhibitor preferentially targets the 2G allele. This was confirmed in transient transfection assays with MMP-1 promoter constructs linked to luciferase. Expression of 2G promoter DNA was 5 – 10X greater than 1G DNA in either cell type, indicating that both melanoma lines contain the appropriate transcription factors necessary to drive expression of the 2G allele, and that the 2G allele is preferentially expressed.

We then studied the paracrine effect of tumor cells on MMP-1 expression in normal stromal cells. We used Northern analysis and real-time RT-PCR to demonstrate that serum-free conditioned medium taken from the A2058 cells could induce MMP-1 expression in normal human foreskin fibroblasts (HFFs), a model for stromal cells. We also used real-time RT-PCR to measure basal and bFGF-induced (10 ng/ml) MMP-1 mRNA in HFFs, which had been genotyped for the SNP. As expected, basal expression was low in all cells, but bFGF gave a 40-fold increase in 1G-containing cells, and an 80-fold increase in 2G cells. Thus, bFGF preferentially stimulates the 2G allele in stromal cells to increase MMP-1 mRNA.

Lastly, we investigated the incidence of the 2G allele in patients with metastatic melanoma. We genotyped 58 patients with metastatic disease. Of these, 30 were heterozygotes and of those, 12 had undergone Loss of Heterozygosity at the MMP-1 locus, 11q 22-23. Ten had retained the 2G allele, with only 2 patients retaining the 1G allele ($P < 0.04$). Since loss of either allele is a random event, we concluded that retention of the 2G allele favors metastasis, which is manifested by metastatic melanomas with the 2G genotype. Therefore, our data show that (a) bFGF production by melanoma cells induces MMP-1 in the tumor cells and in the surrounding stroma, (b) higher levels of MMP-1 are seen in cells with the 2G allele, and (c) the 2G allele can enhance the metastatic potential of melanoma.

T-1

TD-1 WORKSHOP ON CA125; EPITOPES ON RECOMBINANT CA125 REPEAT

Kjell Nustad, MD, PhD, Kari H. Olsen, John B. Beard, PhD, Timothy J. O'Brien, MD, PhD, David J. Warren, PhD
Norwegian Radium Hospital, Montebello, N-0310 Oslo, Norway; University of Arkansas for Medical Sciences, Little Rock, AK

One of the 60 repeats present in CA125 (O'Brien et al., Tumor Biol. 2001; 22: 348-366) was expressed in E. coli as inclusion bodies. The His-tagged repeat was dissolved in urea, purified on a Ni-column, and renatured by dialysis and collected in Tris-buffered saline with various additives. The protein with a predicted 156 amino acids and a MW of 17 200 gave the expected size when analysed by SDS PAGE. However, most preparations formed aggregates of various sizes in native PAGE or gel filtration. These aggregates could not be dissolved by non ionic detergents or high concentration of salt, but were readily reversed by addition of small amounts of SDS. The effect of SDS is strongly influenced by other proteins added.

The same repeat was expressed using a baculovirus approach. The product of the insect cell will be compared with the bacterial product.

Under optimized conditions the repeat behaves very much like intact CA125 in an two-site immunometric assay. Like CA125 this repeat loose epitopes by reduction and alkylation. Previous workshops found that antibodies to CA125 could be grouped as OC125-like antibodies, M11-like antibodies and OV197-like antibodies. The repeat contains the epitopes recognized by all major groups, and all subgroups tested so fare.

The binding of antibodies to the repeat will be analysed using a BiaCore system (Amerham Pharmacia, Biosciences). This will allow measurements of affinities and on- and off-rates.

T-2

TD-10 WORKSHOP ON SQUAMOUS CELL CARCINOMA ANTIGEN; EPITOPES RECOGNIZED BY 13 MONOCLONAL ANTIBODIES

Kjell Nustad, MD, PhD, Tone Varaas, Kari H. Olsen, Elisabeth Paus, PhD
Norwegian Radium Hospital, Montebello, Oslo, Norway

The antigens used to characterize the monoclonal antibodies were recombinant rSCCA1 and rSCCA2 distributed with the antibodies. In addition partly purified SCCA1 and SCCA2 were obtained from tumor extract and saliva by ion exchange chromatography on Mono-S (Ammersham Pharmacia, Biosciences). The proteins were identified by in-house assays specific for SCCA1, SCCA2 and all forms of SCCA.

Binding of radio-labeled recombinant SCCA1 and SCCA2 was used to classify the antibodies in three groups specific for rSCCA1, rSCCA2 or both proteins. These studies were also used to estimate relative affinities of all antibodies for the recombinant proteins. The specificity of the binding to the recombinant proteins was confirmed by inhibition using native SCCA proteins.

Complete cross-inhibition experiments were done using radio-labeled rSCCA1 and rSCCA2, antibody coated on microtiter plates, and inhibiting antibodies used in 100x molar excess over catcher antibodies. Cross-inhibition with native SCCA1 and SCCA2 will also be done.

Immunoradiometric assay combinations were established using all antibodies as catchers and tracer antibodies with native SCCA1 and SCCA2 as analytes.

T-3

TD-8 (CEA) WORKSHOP REPORT

Ole P. Børmer, MD, PhD, Sten Hammarström, PhD, Professor, Bjerner Johan, MD, Yuri Lebedin, MD, Laurent Bellanger, PhD, Masahide Kuroki, MD, PhD, Professor, Jean-Pierre Mach, MD, PhD, John E. Shively, MD, PhD, Tone Varaas, Kjell Nustad, MD, PhD
Central Lab., Norwegian Radium Hospital, Oslo, Norway, Division of Immunology, Umeå University, Umeå, Sweden, Xema-Medica Co., Moscow, Russia, CIS bio international, Bagnols-sur-Ceze, France, Department of Biochemistry, Fukuoka University Medical School, Fukuoka, Japan, Institute of Biochemistry, University of Lausanne, Lausanne, Switzerland, Division of Immunology, City of Hope, Duarte, CA

We previously demonstrated that the down-regulation of c-Myc protein expression in M14 melanoma cells increases the susceptibility to cisplatin [cis-diamminedichloroplatinum(II), (CDDP)] and to a novel anticancer drug ecteinascidin-743 (ET-743). Since the decreased c-Myc expression is associated with a concomitant reduction in the human Telomerase Reverse Transcriptase (hTERT) expression and telomerase activity, telomere shortening and dysfunction, the aim of this study was to investigate the role of telomerase function on the ability of c-Myc to modulate the CDDP and ET-743 sensitivity. Reconstitution of hTERT in the c-Myc low-expressing clones restores telomerase activity, reduces telomere dysfunction, and decreases the sensitivity to both drugs. The reduced sensitivity to CDDP and ET-743 is due to the ability of cells to recover from drug-induced damage. Reactivation of telomere function modifies cell cycle progression, enabling the cells to recover from drug-induced G2/M block and consequently protecting them from apoptosis. Taken together these results open the possibility to use c-myc antisense, able to induce telomere dysfunction, followed by telomerase inhibitors and CDDP/ET-743 treatment, to improve the chemotherapeutic response of melanoma.

Supported by grants from Italian Association for Cancer Research (A.I.R.C.), Ministero della Sanità, and CNR-MIUR.

T-4

CHARACTERISATION OF ISOBM TD-10 SCCA MONOCLONAL ANTIBODIES

Olle Nilsson, PhD, Eva Röijer, PhD, Karin Nilsson
CanAg Diagnostics AB, Majnabbeterminalen, Gothenburg, Sweden

Squamous cell carcinoma antigen (SCCA) is a serological marker for squamous cell carcinomas (SCC) of the uterine cervix, lung, head and neck, vulva, and esophagus. Serum concentrations of SCCA in patients with SCC are correlated to the clinical stage, tumour volume and to the degree of histological differentiation of the tumor; recurrence or progressive disease can be detected several months before clinical evidence [1-3]. SCCA belongs to the serpin family and consists of at least two different proteins that are 92% identical at the amino acid level. SCCA1 inhibits the papain-like cystein proteinases cathepsin S, K, and L while SCCA2 inhibits the chymotrypsin-like serine proteinases cathepsin G and Mast Cell Chymase [4, 5].

In the ISOBM TD-10 Workshop on SCC antigen the monoclonal antibodies ISOBM 347-359 were characterized. Reactivity with recombinant SCCA1 and SCCA2 antigen was determined in ELISA's. Competitive inhibition and determination of dose-response in sandwich immunoassays as well as reactivity with different recombinant SCC antigens were determined for epitope mapping. The reactivity of the different ISOBM SCC MAb's with active serpin and/or serpin complex was determined in assays using Cathepsin G and Cathepsin L as target proteases.

1. Snyderman, C.H., et al., A reappraisal of the squamous cell carcinoma antigen as a tumor marker in head and neck cancer. Arch Otolaryngol Head Neck Surg, 1995. 121(11): p. 1294-7.
2. de Bruijn, H.W., et al., The clinical value of squamous cell carcinoma antigen in cancer of the uterine cervix. Tumour Biol, 1998. 19(6): p. 505-16.
3. Kato, H., Squamous Cell Carcinoma Antigen, in Serological Cancer Markers, S. Sell, Editor. 1992, The Humana Press: Totowa, NJ. p. 437-451.
4. Schick, C., et al., The reactive site loop of the serpin SCCA1 is essential for cysteine proteinase inhibition. Proc Natl Acad Sci U S A, 1998. 95(23): p. 13465-70.
5. Luke, C., et al., Simple modifications of the serpin reactive site loop convert SCCA2 into a cysteine proteinase inhibitor: a critical role for the P3' proline in facilitating RSL cleavage. Biochemistry, 2000. 39(24): p. 7081-91.

T-5

NON-CA125 MONOCLONAL ANTIBODIES SPECIFICALLY RECOGNIZE RECOMBINANT CA125 – SUGGESTED SPECIFICITY AGAINST CA125-RELATED CARBOHYDRATE ANTIGEN(S)

Yuri Lebedin, Sergey Prokofiev
Xema-Medica Co.Ltd., Moscow, Russia

Monoclonal antibodies X81 and X3LE were raised against highly glycosylated mucin prepared from gastric carcinoma tissue containing CA125 along with high proportion of CA72-4 (sT/sTn) antigen. These mAbs show low to negligible inhibition of all TD1 (CA125) workshop mAbs suggesting the specificity different from CA125. In sandwich EIAs with epitope B CA125 mAbs, both antibodies shown positive signals in patient sera in absence of 'regular' CA125. However, in immunoblotting with natural CA125 preparations, both mAbs show the staining pattern identical to CA125 mAbs. In addition, both mAbs bind recombinant CA125 (rCA) preparation obtained from T.O'Brien (University of Arkansas) though the degree of binding is considerably lower than expected according to its CA125 content. Both X81 and X3LE slightly stained rCA preparation in immunoblotting. Neuraminidase treatment partly abolished binding of X81 but not X3LE to rCA; trypsin treatment fully abolished binding of both mAbs. We concluded that two mAbs may recognize CA125-related carbohydrate epitope which is weakly expressed by partly processed recombinant antigen.

T-6

COMPARATIVE SCREENING FOR HUMAN AUTOANTIBODIES AGAINST RECOMBINANT CA125 REPEAT ANTIGEN AND PURIFIED NATURAL OVARIAN CARCINOMA MUCIN

Yuri Lebedin, Larisa Blidchenko, Maya Zhdanovich
Xema-Medica Co.Ltd., Moscow, Russia

Recombinant CA125 repeat (rCA) was obtained from T.O'Brien (University of Arkansas); natural ovarian carcinoma mucin antigen lot CA23 was purified from single patient ascitic fluid and contained high CA125 activity (>100 kiloUnits per mg). Sera of 85 autoimmune patients (rheumatoid arthritis, SLE, Sjogren syndrome), and 360 randomly selected patients were tested for presence of anti-rCA and anti-CA23 by solid phase EIA. A correlation between two antigen measurements reached considerable level ($r=0.43$) though was not statistically significant ($p>0.1$). Eight sera shown clear positivity to both rCA and CA23 (group 1); two sera were positive only for rCA (group 2); and 18 sera were positive only for CA23 (group 3). All group 1 (double positive) and group 2 (rCA positive) sera shown weak to moderate signal in EIA; none of these sera shown visible bands in immunoblotting on corresponding antigens. Among 18 group 3 sera (CA23 positive), 12 sera shown clear band in HMW zone of immunoblotting (>500 kDa). Affinity purified human anti-CA23 antibodies from high titer donor plasma did not recognize rCA. We suggest that CA125 repeat determinant can induce at least spontaneous antibody response in humans though the degree of this response is low and there is possibility of detecting false response to the impurities. From other side, natural ovarian mucin is shown to contain non-CA125 HMW autoantigen(s) of presently unknown nature.

T-7

TD-10 SQUAMOUS CELL CARCINOMA ANTIGEN WORKSHOP

Sule Cataltepe, MD, Cliff J Luke, PhD, Gary A Silverman, MD, PhD
Children's Hospital, Harvard Medical School, Boston, MA

Method: A total of 520 ng of rSCCA1, rSCCA2, recombinant serpinB12 and chicken ovalbumin were separated by SDS-PAGE and electroblotted at 100V for 1 hr onto nitrocellulose membranes. Each membrane was cut into 13 equal-sized strips that contained 40 ng protein. After three rinses in wash buffer (PBS, pH 7.4, 0.1% Tween-20), the blots were incubated for 1 h in 5% dry milk in wash buffer. Sets of four strips containing ovalbumin, serpin B12, SCCA1 and SCCA2 were incubated with each one of the purified SCCA antibodies at a 0.004 mg/ml concentration, diluted in 1% dry milk/wash buffer. The membranes were washed three times in wash buffer, and then incubated with peroxidase-conjugated goat anti-mouse IgG as the secondary antibody. After 3 rinses in wash buffer, the blots were incubated for 5 min with chemiluminiscent detection kit, ECL (Amersham Pharmacia). Chemiluminescence was detected by autoradiography.

Results: None of the antibodies showed a cross-reaction with chicken ovalbumin or recombinant serpin B12. Mouse anti-SCCA antibodies #347, 348, 349, 351, 355 and 366 did not react with either rSCCA1 or rSCCA2. Antibodies #350, 352, 354 and 359 reacted only with rSCCA1. One antibody, #357, reacted both with rSCCA1 and rSCCA2. Antibody #353 was the only SCCA2-specific antibody.

T-8

HETEROGENEITY OF SQUAMOUS CELL CARCINOMA ANTIGEN DEMONSTRATED BY TWO-DIMENSIONAL ELECTROPHORESIS

Yoshinori Suminami, MD, Shugo Nawata, MD, Hiroshi Hirakawa, MD, Fumitaka Numa, MD, Hiroshi Kato, MD
Yamaguchi University, Ube, Japan

Two homologous serpins, squamous cell carcinoma (SCC) antigen-1 and -2 in tumor tissue have been identified by two-dimensional electrophoresis (2-DE) combined with immunoblotting using specific antibodies for SCC antigen (Mab13, Mab27). Namly, SCC antigen-1 was separated into four spots with pI 6.4-5.9 and Mr 44 500-45 000 including the phosphorylated form, while SCC antigen-2 was detected as three spots with pI 5.7-5.5 and Mr 44 500. By nondenaturing 2-DE, we also found that all spots of SCC antigen-2 were detected as polymeric forms, which were recognized by Mab27, but not Mab13. These results indicated that there are several forms of both SCC antigens in vivo. In the present study, we examined the immunoreactivity of the latest antibodies (8H11, 10C12) against native SCC antigen from the view of its molecular heterogeneity. 8H11 antibody detected main spot of SCC antigen-1 with pI 6.4, but not phosphorylated SCC antigen-1 with pI 5.9, indicating that 8H11-associated epitope are located at the phosphorylated site on SCC antigen-1. On the other hand, 10C12 antibody detected all three spots of SCC antigen-2 even if they were polymerized in native state. Furthermore, we will report the serum levels of SCC antigen-1and SCC antigen-2 in patients bearing cervical cancer by the discriminatory ELISA using these specific antibody, and discuss the necessity to discriminate SCC antigen-1 and SCC antigen-2 which have the different biological function.

O-1

MOUSE MODELS OF IMPAIRED SPERMATOGENESIS; RELEVANCE TO UNDERSTANDING TESTICULAR MALIGNANCIES

José Luis Millán, PhD
The Burnham Institute, La Jolla, CA

Spermatogenesis is a complex process by which postmeiotic male germ cells differentiate into mature spermatozoa. Differentiating male germ cells often express testis-specific transcripts, isozymes and molecules. One such example is the cytochrome c (Cyt cT) gene distinct from the cytochrome c expressed in somatic cells (Cyt cS). To examine the role of Cyt cT in the germ cells, we generated mice null for Cyt cT1. Homozygous Cyt cT -/- pups were statistically under-represented (21%) but develop normally and are fertile. However, spermatozoa isolated from cauda epididymis of Cyt cT null animals are less effective in fertilizing oocytes in vitro and contain reduced levels of ATP than wild-type sperm. Cyt cT null mice often exhibit early atrophy of the testes after 4 months of age, losing germ cells as a result of increased apoptosis. However, no difference in the activation of caspase-3, -8 or -9 was observed between the Cyt cT -/- testes and controls indicating that this apoptosis is not mediated by caspases. At all stages of spermatogenic maturation, Sertoli cells and germ cells communicate through direct cell-cell adhesion and paracrine stimulation. Despite our understanding of these cell types, the mechanisms that mediate adhesive interaction between Sertoli and germ cells remain unknown. We found that following a targeted disruption of a gene encoding the Golgi alpha-mannosidase IIx (MX) male offspring were infertile due to inefficient spermatogenesis2. Testes from MX-deficient males were smaller than those from heterozygous and wild type littermates, and exhibited reduction of spermatozoa. Both the morphology of the testis and in vitro Sertoli -germ cell adhesion assays indicated a failure in adhesion between Sertoli cells and spermatocytes. We were able to identify a carbohydrate structure, which is unique to the testis, that specifically inhibits Sertoli-germ cell adhesion through a receptor with binding affinities similar to that of the GSA II lectin. Understanding the apoptotic regulation of germ cells and their interaction with Sertoli cells is important to elucidate the pathogenesis of testicular germ cell tumors (TGCTs). Seminomas and nonseminomas represent the invasive stages of TGCTs, characterized by extra copies of the short arm of chromosome 12. We have demonstrated that a novel gene, defender-against-apoptotic cell death-R (DAD-R), is amplified in TGCTs and that DAD-R maps closely to the centromeric breakpoint of the 12p amplicon3. Elevated DAD-R expression in seminomas and nonseminomas correlates with invasive growth and a reduced level of apoptosis associated with an earlier clinical onset. Furthermore, GSAII lectin staining of germ cell tumor and human fetal testis correlates well with the germ cells interaction with Sertoli cells.

1Narisawa et al. Mol. Cell Biol. In Press (2002)
2Akama et al. Science 296: 124-127 (2002)
3Zafarana et al. Cancer Res. 62: 1822-1831 (2002)

O-2

DIFFERENTIAL INVOLVEMENT OF THE HYPERMETHYLATOR PHENOTYPE IN HEREDITARY AND SPORADIC COLORECTAL CANCERS WITH HIGH-FREQUENCY MICROSATELLITE INSTABILITY

Shina Horiuchi, MD, Hiroyuki Yamamoto, MD, PhD, Yongfen Min, MD, PhD, Yasushi Adachi, MD, PhD, Mio Yoshida, Katsuhiko Nosho, Hiroaki Taniguchi, Akravit Vinitketkumnuen, Fumio Itoh, MD, PhD, Kohzoh Imai, MD, PhD
First Department of Internal Medicine, Sapporo Medical University
Sapporo, Japan

High-frequency microsatellite instability (MSI-H) due to defective DNA mismatch repair occurs in the majority of hereditary non-polyposis colorectal cancers and in a subset of sporadic malignant tumors. Clinicopathologic and genotypic features of MSI-H colorectal tumors in hereditary nonpolyposis colorectal cancer (HNPCC) patients and those in sporadic cases are very similar, but not identical. Correlation between the MSI phenotype and aberrant DNA methylation has recently been highlighted. A strong association between MSI and CpG island methylation has been well characterized in sporadic colorectal cancers with MSI-H, but not in those of hereditary origin. To address the issue, we analyzed hereditary and sporadic colorectal cancers for aberrant DNA methylation of target genes using methylation-specific polymerase chain reaction. DNA methylation of the hMLH1, p16INK4A, O-6-methylguanine DNA methyltransferase (MGMT), thrombospondin-1, retinoic acid receptor beta, adenomatous polyposis coli, and p14ARF genes was found in 0%, 23%, 10%, 3%, 73%, 53%, and 33% of 30 MSI-H cancers in HNPCC patients and in 80%, 55%, 23%, 23%, 58%, 35%, and 50% of 40 sporadic colorectal cancers with MSI-H, respectively. Cases showing methylation at 3 or more loci of 6 genes other than hMLH1 were defined as CpG island methylator phenotype-positive (CIMP+), and 23% of HNPCC tumors and 53% of sporadic cancers with MSI-H were CIMP+ (P = 0.018). Differences in the extent of CpG island methylation, coupled with the differential involvement of several genes by methylation, in HNPCC tumors and sporadic MSI-H colorectal cancers may be associated with diverging developmental pathways in hereditary and sporadic cancers despite similar MSI-H phenotypes.

O-3

LABYRINTHIN IS A MUTATED FORM OF JUNCTIN/JUNCTATE ASSOCIATED WITH THE HUMAN ADENOCARCINOMA PHENOTYPE

J.A. Radosevich, B. Bentz, G.K. Haines, III
ImmvaRx, Inc., Rockford, IL, Memorial Sloan Kettering, New York, NY, Northwestern University, Chicago, IL

Junctin is a normal cellular protein which is bound to calsequestrin in cardiac and skeletal muscle, and is a key factor in regulating the intracellular free calcium levels within cells. Several isoforms of Junctin, including Junctate, have been found in normal cells. As transmembrane proteins, Junctin/Junctate is firmly anchored in the lipid bilayer, and have the sarco(endo)plasmic reticulum molecular signal to target Junctin/Junctate to remain in that cellular organelle. Labyrinthin, has been studied for all most two decades, and has been shown to be over expressed in human adenocarcinomas arising throughout the human body. This cell surface oncofetal protein has been used as a target for both radiolabeled and chemotherapeutic conjugated mouse monoclonal antibodies to locate and selective kill positively expressing human adenocarcinoma cells lines both in vivo and in vitro. Labyrinthin expression has been shown to be modulated in response to changes in intracellular free calcium levels similar to that of Junctin/Junctate. Sense/Anti-Sense Labyrinthin experiments demonstrate that Labyrinthin confers the Adenocarcinoma phenotype to human fibroblasts, and that human Adenocarcinoma cells require the expression of this gene. Sequence analysis of these and other related genes support the hypothesis that Labyrinthin is a mutated form of Junctin/Junctate, which due to the loss of the sarco(endo)plasmic reticulum targeting signal, results in altered intracellular free calcium levels and the adenocarcinoma phenotype. The lack of the sarco(endo)plasmic reticulum targeting signal offers a mechanism by which this normally sequestered intracellular protein (in normal cells) becomes abundantly expressed in the cell surface of human Adenocarcinomas. These data support the approach of targeting Labyrinthin with humanized monoclonal antibodies and as a target for a pan-Adenocarcinoma cancer vaccine.

O-4

EXPRESSION OF GENES INVOLVED IN THE OESTRADIOL METABOLIC AND SIGNALLING PATHWAYS IN TUMOURS FROM BREAST CANCER PATIENTS TREATED WITH NEOADJUVANT AROMATASE INHIBITOR ANASTROZOLE

Vessela N. Kristensen, PhD, Jürgen Geisler, MD, PhD, Noriko Yoshimura, MD, Nobuhiro Harada, MD, PhD, Ole Christian Lingjærde, PhD, Per Eystein Lønning, MD, PhD, Anne-Lise Børresen-Dale, PhD
Department of Genetics, Norwegian Radium Hospital, Oslo, Norway; Department of Oncology, Haukeland Hospital, Bergen, Norway; Department of Biochemistry, Fujita Health University, Japan; Institute of Informatics, University of Oslo, Norway

Twelve postmenopausal women with locally advanced breast cancer (mean age 67) received anastrozole (Arimidex®) as an oral dose of 1mg once daily for 15 weeks prior to surgery. Quantitative analysis of intratumoral mRNA was performed before and after the treatment for the following genes: aromatase (CYP19), 17-b hydroxysteroid dehydrogenase I and II (HSDI and HSDII), steroid sulfatase (STS), oestrone sulfotransferase (EST) as well as for oestrogen receptor (ESR-a and ESR-b), cyclin D1 (CYCLD1) and cErbB2(ERBB2/HER2). mRNA expression data for CYP19, HSDI,II and EST/STS were correlated to intratumoural levels of their substrates: oestrone (E1), oestradiol (E2) and oestrone sulfate (E1S), before and after the treatment. While the levels of some transcripts remained basically unchanged (HSDI and II) before and after the treatment, others were dramatically increased (STS, CYP19) or decreased (EST) and this behaviour differed in the different response groups. There was a strong correlation between the expression of mRNA of STS and EST ($r= 0.995$, $p<0,0001$). Levels of CYP19 (aromatase) mRNA correlated to the amounts of E2 before but not after the treatment when the EST mRNA levels appeared to be in correlation to E2 ($r=0,626$, $p<0.029$). There was an inverse correlation between the expression of HSDII mRNA and the levels of E2 both before and after the treatment. The decrease of E1 and E2 as a result of aromatase inhibition inversely correlated to an increase in EST mRNA levels ($r=-0.745$, $p<0,005$). An increase of levels of mRNA of aromatase in patients with partial response (PR) ($n=3$) was observed. mRNA of aromatase on the contrary was decreased in PD ($n=2$)patients after treatment.

O-5

IDENTIFICATION OF NOVEL TUMOR SUPPRESSOR GENES BY A NOVEL GENOME SCREENING TECHNIQUE, METHYLATED CPG ISLAND AMPLIFICATION

Minoru Toyota, MD, PhD, Fumio Itoh, MD, PhD, Hiromu Suzuki, MD, PhD, Kazuhiro Ogi, MD, PhD, Toshiro Obata, MD, PhD, Ayumi Satoh, MD, PhD, Kimishige Akino, MD, PhD, Takashi Tokino, MD, PhD, Kohzoh Imai, MD, PhD
Sapporo Medical University, Sapporo, Japan

Evidence now suggests that transcriptional silencing of selected genes by DNA methylation plays a crucial role in the development and progression of human cancer. To isolate genes inactivated by hypermethylation in human cancer, we have applied a PCR-based methylation screening technique, CpG island amplification (MCA). Using amplicon prepared from cancer cell lines as a tester and amplicon from normal tissue as a driver, we have isolated 400 sequences hypermethylated in various type of human cancers including, colorectal, gastric, head and neck and prostate cancers. Of these, 210 clones fulfill the criteria of CpG islands. The clones include several genes previously reported for hypermethylation in various human tumors, PAX-2, PAX-7, and progesteron receptor, indicating that MCA is an efficient method to isolate genes hypermethylated in cancer. One of the clones was matched to the genomic sequence obtained by human genome project. An open reading frame was predicted using exon prediction program and EST data base search. Sequences were verified with RT-PCR analysis followed by DNA sequences. This gene, named MIMC1 (methylated in multiple cancer 1), is methylated in 2 of 10 OSCC cell lines, 4 of 10 colorectal cancer cell lines, and 5 of 15 gastric cancer cell lines, but was not methylated in normal tongue tissues and normal colon mucosa. Dense methylation of 5' region of the gene was closely associated with loss of expression, and expression was restored by treatment of methyltransferase inhibitor, 5-aza-dC, indicating that aberrant methylation of MIMC1 is responsible for gene silencing. Chromatin immunoprecipitation using anti acetylated histone H3 and H4 revealed that histone deacetylation plays a role in methylation dependent gene silencing of MIMC1. These data indicated that the clones identified by MCA are useful molecular markers to identify novel genes inactivated by hypermethylation in human cancer.

O-6

PHOSPHORYLATION OF CEACAM1-4S IN TRANSFECTED MCF-7 MAMMARY CARCINOMA CELLS INDUCES LUMEN FORMATION BY APOPTOSIS

John E. Shively, PhD, Julia Kirshner, BS, Charng Jui Chen, PhD, Detlef Schumann, PhD, Mark Sherman, PhD
City of Hope, Duarte, CA

The cell-cell adhesion molecule carcinoembryonic antigen cell adhesion molecule 1 (CEACAM1) is a cell surface glycoprotein and a member of the CEA gene family. Normal mammary epithelial cells express CEACAM1 in a polarized, lumenal orientation and CEACAM1 has been shown to play an essential role in lumen formation in a mammary morphogenesis model using MCF10F cells. Here we show that MCF7 mammary carcinoma cells, which do not express CEACAM1 or make lumens when grown in Matrigel, are restored to a normal morphogenic program when transfected with CEACAM1-4S, the short cytoplasmic isoform of CEACAM1 with four Ig-like extracellular domains. Specific staining with anti-cytokeratin 18 antibody M30 or MitoSensor dye demonstrated that the lumens are formed by apoptosis of the central cells within the alveolar structures. Moreover, apoptotic cells within the lumen were the same cells that expressed CEACAM1-4S, as demonstrated by visualization of CEACAM1-4S-exoGFP fusion protein expressed in MCF7 cells together with MitoSensor staining. Furthermore cells undergoing lumen formation in Matrigel test positive for phospho Ser/Thr on immunoprecipitated CEACAM1-4S. Since residues Thr423 and Ser425 in the cytoplasmic domain are putative protein kinase C phosphorylation sites, we mutated these residues to Asp or Ala conferring pseudophosphorylation and null mutations respectively. MCF7 cells transfected with the Ala null mutants (T423A, S425A, and T423A,S425A) did not form lumens in Matrigel. In contrast, the T423D mutation lead to colony death for cells grown in Matrigel but not on plastic. Strikingly, the T423D,S425D double mutation was lethal even for MCF7 or Hela cells grown on plastic, with cell death occurring as early as 24 hours post transfection. Transfection of MCF7 cells with CEACAM1-4L, the long cytoplasmic isoform of CEACAM1 with four extracellular Ig-like domains, resulted in massive death of these cells when grown in Matrigel but not on plastic. These data suggest that both isoforms are capable of delivering a death signal, but CEACAM1-4S, the predominant isoform in normal mammary epithelial cells, is probably the physiologically relevant isoform for these cells. Taken together these data demonstrate that CEACAM1-4S can revert tumor cells to a normal morphogenic program by promoting apoptosis of the cells in the center of the acini that lack contact with the extracellular matrix.

O-7

JADE-1, A NOVEL PHD PROTEIN STABILIZED BY VHL THAT MAY PARTICIPATE IN RENAL TUMOR SUPPRESSION

Mi Zhou, PhD, Hongmei Wang, MS, Jonathan J. Ross, Rebecca L. Foy, Herbert T. Cohen, MD
Department of Medicine, Boston University Medical Center, Boston, MA

The von Hippel-Lindau (VHL) gene is the major renal cancer gene in adults. However, the mechanism by which VHL protein acts as a renal tumor suppressor remains unknown. To identify low-occupancy VHL interactors that might have relevance to renal cancer, we screened an adult human kidney library against human VHL in a yeast 2-hybrid approach and have identified a novel, strong VHL-interactor. We call this gene (and protein) Jade-1 (gene for Apoptosis and Differentiation in Epithelia. Jade-1 protein is short-lived and contains a candidate destabilizing (PEST) domain and plant homeodomain (PHD) motifs, which are not required for the VHL interaction. Jade-1 protein expression is highest in renal cancer precursors, the proximal tubule cells, and correlates positively with their differentiation. Jade-1 protein is expressed in cytoplasm and the nucleus diffusely and in speckles, where it partly colocalizes with VHL. VHL reintroduction into renal cancer cells increases endogenous Jade-1 protein abundance up to 10-fold. Moreover, VHL increases Jade-1 protein half-life up to 3-fold. Intriguingly, in early studies, renal cancer-associated VHL truncation and substitution mutations are unable to increase Jade-1 protein stability. In contrast, naturally-occurring VHL mutations that do not confer renal cancer risk, such as the Y98H and Y112H mutations, stabilize Jade-1 protein as well as wild-type VHL. Functionally, Jade-1 inhibits growth of renal cells. Jade-1 overexpression causes apoptosis, and generation of stable Jade-1 overexpressing renal cancer cell lines has been far less successful than VHL-overexpressing lines. Thus, direct protein stabilization is identified as a new VHL function. Furthermore, Jade-1 protein represents a novel, growth-inhibiting candidate regulatory factor that may be important in VHL-mediated renal tumor suppression.

O-9

ALPHA-FETOPROTEIN ACTIVATES APOPTOSIS IN TUMOR CELLS VIA INDUCTION OF THE CYTOCHROME C RELEASE AND POSITIVE REGULATION OF CYTOCHROME C-DEPENDED CASPASE ACTIVATION

Elena I. Dudich, PhD, Lidia N. Semenkova, PhD, Igor V. Dudich, PhD, Natalia A. Tokhtamisheva, PhD, Timo K. Korpela, PhD, Prof., Juan-Antonio Palop-Cubillo, PhD, Prof.
Institute of Immunological Engineering Lyubuchany, Russia; Turku University, Finland; University of Navarra, Spain

Previous results have shown that oncoembryonic marker α-fetoprotein (AFP) is able to induce apoptosis in tumor cells through activation of caspase-3 bypassing Fas and TNFR-dependent signaling. We show here that AFP can directly induce apoptosis by activation of intracellular death-machinery without membrane receptor-mediated clustering or signals. AFP-treatment of tumor cells induces fast release of cytochrome c (cyt-c) from mitochondria. In a cell free system, AFP regulates caspase-9 and -3 activation diversely: AFP enhances the effects of suboptimal doses of cyt-c and suppresses the effects mediated by high doses of cyt-c. AFP was unable to induce caspase-9 and caspase-3 activation and processing in a cell-free system in the absence of cyt-c while AFP significantly enhanced caspase processing in the presence of endogenous or exogenous cyt-c. AFP was unable to directly activate isolated procaspase-3 immobilized on the agarose beads, demonstrating a requirement for a presence of additional adapter factors. A series of immunodepletion experiments demonstrated that a presence in cell extracts of the main apoptosome-forming proteins: cyt-c, dATP, caspase-9 and caspase-3 as well as of some other adapter proteins, is required for AFP-mediated triggering of apoptosis. Chromatographic analysis of the apoptosome assembly formed in the cell-free extracts in the presence of AFP demonstrated that AFP positively regulates cytochrome c/dATP-mediated apoptosome complex formation and stimulates recruitment of caspases and Apaf-1 into the complex. Our data suggest that AFP may regulate cell death by displacing of cIAP-2, the inhibitor-of-apoptosis-protein, from the apoptosome resulting in promoting of caspase-3 activation and release from the complex.

O-10

A COMPARATIVE ANALYSIS OF BIOLOGICAL EFFECT OF HUMAN AFP AND SYNTHETIC PEPTIDE (AFP 13-19) ON THE ACTIVATION PROCESS IN LYMPHOCYTES

Alexander N. Kazimirsky, MD, PhD, Jean M. Salmasy, MD, PhD, Alexander A. Terentiev, MD, PhD, Gennadij V. Poryadin, MD, PhD, Yurij S. Tatarinov, MD, PhD
Russian State Medical University, Moscow, Russia

The biological screening of peptide fragments of AFP molecule enable us to carry out this protein molecule structural and functional analysis. Development of a pathological activation of immune system leading to overproduction of IgE lies in the basis of the pathogenesis of such human diseases as bronchial asthma, atopic dermatitis and pollinosis. A study of the influence of human alpha-fetoprotein (AFP) and synthetic peptide (AFP13-19) on the lymphocytes of 6 patients with atopic bronchial asthma in the acute period of the disease was made. The lymphocytes of these patients present a cell model of an intensive activation process of the lymphocytes, developing in the direction of formation of highly differentiated shapes of B-cells and characterized by dysfunction of activating apoptosis. We were defining the quantity of the lymphocytes expressing the following line of antigens: CD3, CD4, CD8, CD16, CD56, CD20, CD72, CD38, CD23, CD25, CD71, HLA-DR, CD95, CD54, mIgM, mIgG, l- and k- chain of the immunoglobulins. The cultivation of the lymphocytes, received from patients, was done during 16 hours in the presence of AFP with its final concentration of 5 mg/ml or synthetic peptide AFP13-19 with concentration of 10-8 M. Two immunotropic effects are observed under the influence of AFP. The first consists of an authentic decrease of markers of activation B-lymphocytes (CD23), as well as markers of early and late activation lymphocytes CD25, CD71 and HLA-DR. The second biological effect of AFP consists in an increase of the quantity of the lymphocytes expressing the receptor of the activation apoptosis CD95. Synthetic peptide AFP13-19 doesn't influence the expression of the early activation antigens (CD25 and CD71), but causes a considerable increase of cell quantity, positively in expressing to the activation apoptosis receptors. At the same time the quantity of the lymphocytes, carrying the receptors of the late differentiated state (HLA-DR+-cells), considerably reduced. Thus, it's possible to conclude that a molecule of AFP has in its composition a few peptide successions with various immunotropic effects. The initial part of the protein chain of AFP, as our results show, is able to strengthen the induction of the activation apoptosis of the lymphocytes promoting the maintenance of immune tolerance.

O-11

IDENTIFICATION OF THE MAJOR CK2 PHOSPHORYLATION SITE IN BETA-CATENIN AND ITS ROLE IN BETA-CATENIN FUNCTION

Diane Song, PhD, Isabel Dominguez, PhD, Junko Mizumo, Esther Landesman-Bollag, PhD, Maurya Kaut, Scott Mohr, PhD, David Seldin, MD, PhD
Boston University Medical Center
Boston, MA

Protein kinase CK2 is a ubiquitously expressed serine/threonine kinase involved in many biological processes. It is overexpressed in many malignancies including rodent and human breast cancer, and transgenic expression of CK2 in the mammary gland of mice promotes breast cancer. Transgenic CK2 tumors frequently upregulate beta-catenin, the critical transcriptional cofactor in the Wnt signaling pathway. CK2 is upregulated in Wnt-transfected mammary epithelial cells, and it can be found in a complex with dishevelled (a Wnt signaling intermediate) and beta-catenin. Beta-catenin is a substrate for CK2 and inhibition of CK2 reduces levels of beta-catenin and dishevelled. CK2 prevents proteasomal degradation of beta-catenin and potentiates beta-catenin-dependent LEF-1 transcriptional activity. The major phosphorylation site on beta-catenin is threonine 393; mutation of this site reduces beta-catenin co-transcriptional activity and protein stability. Thus, one mechanism of CK2-induced transformation is potentiation of Wnt signaling through stabilization of the critical beta-catenin transcriptional cofactor, and CK2 may play a physiological role in Wnt signaling.

O-12

INVOLVEMENT OF CASEIN KINASE I (CKI)-EPSILON IN CELL DIFFERENTIATION INTO GRANULOCYTES

Toshimitsu Matsui, MD, PhD, Atsuo Okamura, MD, Manabu Shimoyama, MD, PhD, Hiroshi Gomyo, MD, Kimikazu Yakushijin, MD, Norinaga Urahama, MD
Hematology/Oncology Division, Department of Medicine, Kobe University Graduate School of Medicine, Kobe, Japan

The gene encoding casein kinase I-epsilon (CKI-e) is widely conserved from yeast to mammals. The human CKI-e gene localized in chromosome 22q12-13 is ubiquitously expressed in various tissues including hematopoietic cells. Although the gene product has been shown to play an important role in DNA repair, cellular morphology and Wnt-signaling, it remains clarified whether the gene is directly involved in carcinogenesis. We found a specific down-regulation of CKI-e expression along myeloid cell differentiation into mature granulocyte. A 46-kDa CKI-e protein in promyelocytic leukemia HL-60 cells was also decreased in company with the retinoic acid-induced terminal differentiation to polymorphonucler cells.

Thus, we studied the functional significance of CKI-e in granulocyte differentiation by introducing CKI-e or kinase-dead CKI-e cDNA into mouse myeloid progenitor, 32D cells using a retrovirus vector. G-CSF or GM-CSF reduced the expression level of CKI-e in 32D cells. Overexpression of CKI-e inhibited the cytokine-induced differentiation into granulocyte, while kinase-dead CKI-e accelerated the differentiation. These results indicate that the expression level of CKI-e regulated by G-CSF or GM-CSF is directly involved in the control cell differentiation into mature granulocytes. It is of interest whether CKI-e is involved in leukomogenesis and could be a molecular target for intervention.

O-13

STRUCTURE-FUNCTION ANALYSIS OF VEGFR-1 AND VEGFR-2: WHAT HAVE WE LEARNED FROM CHIMERA SYSTEM?

Nader Rahimi, PhD, Volken Dayanir, MD, Fredric Majnoun, Rosana D. Meyer, MD
Boston University, School of Medicine, Departments of Ophthalmology and Biochemistry
Boston, MA

Activation of vascular endothelial growth factor receptor-1 & 2 (VEGFR-1 and VEGFR-2) play a critical role in vasculogenesis and angiogenesis. However, the mechanism by which VEGFRs activation elicit these cellular events is not fully understood. We recently have constructed a chimeric receptor containing the extracellular domain of human CSF-1R/c-fms, fused with the entire transmembrane and cytoplasmic domains of murine VEGFR-1 and VEGFR-2. Selective activation of chimeric VEGFR-2, but not VEGFR-1 stimulated endothelial cell growth. Co-expression of chimeric VEGFR-1 and VEGFR-2 suppressed VEGFR-2-mediated endothelial cell growth (Rahimi et al., JBC 275: 16986-16992, 2000). Site-directed mutagenesis demonstrated that tyrosines 799 and 1173 are required for VEGFR-2-mediated endothelial cell growth and activation of PI 3-kinase (Dayanir et al. JBC 276: 17686-17692, 2001). Further site-directed mutagenesis demonstrated a novel role for tyrosine 1212, located in the carboxyl domain of VEGFR-2 (Meyer et al. JBC in Press, 2002). The information obtained from chimeric system suggest that ligand-dependent activation of VEGFR-1 and VEGFR-1 are differentially regulated and tyrosine 1212 in particular and C-terminus of VEGFR-2 in general involved in a novel mechanism to control VEGFR-2 activation and subsequently angiogenesis.

O-14

FUNCTIONAL REQUIREMENT OF AKT ASSOCIATION AND OLIGOMERIZATION FOR THE AKT KINASE COACTIVATOR TCL1

Masa Noguchi, MD, PhD, Larmo Laine, MD, PhD, Gerald Kunstle, PhD, Marc-Henri Stern, MD
Beth Israel Deaconess Medical Center, Boston, MA; Institute Curie, Paris, France

Akt/PKB, a serine-threonine kinase plays a central role in the regulation of cell survival and proliferation. Until recently the function of the TCL1 protooncogene was unknown. We have previously demonstrated that the protooncogene TCL1 is an Akt kinase coactivator. TCL1 binds to Akt via the PH domain and as a result alters its biological activity. TCL1 interaction with Akt, facilitates formation of a high molecular weight protein complex, and activates Akt. Moreover, TCL1 enhanced Akt-dependent cellular proliferation and survival.

Using yeast two-hybrid screen with a random TCL1 fragment library to identify fragments that no longer interact with Akt, we were able to map the domains of TCL1 responsible for Akt association and homodimerization. We have further defined the function of these two domains in the TCL1-induced Akt activation process. TCL1 facilitates the hetero-oligomerization of Akt isoforms and transphosphorylation between the Akt molecules. Our results demonstrate that "non-transmembrane intracellular kinases" like Akt can form hetero-oligomers with TCL1, and, as a consequence enhance their kinase activity via transphosphorylation.

These findings also provide the molecular basis for the survival dynamics of clonal expansion of human T cell prolymphocytic leukemia (T-PLL) in which TCL1 is overexpressed.

O-15

REGULATION OF AIM-1 PROTEIN LEVEL IS IMPORTANT FOR PLOIDY PROMOTION: AN IN VIVO STUDY

Ying Zhang, Guangyao Yu, MD, PhD, Paul Toselli, MD, Carl Jackson, PhD, Katya Ravid, PhD
Boston University School of Medicine, Boston, MA; St.Jude Children, Memphis, Tennessee

The endomitotic cell cycle, involving repeated rounds of DNA replication without cell division, is an essential part of megakaryocytopoiesis. It is also prevalent in other cell types under stress or in cancer. The Mpl-ligand, also known as thrombopoietin (TPO) or megakaryocyte growth and development factor (MGDF), has been shown to regulate and promote endomitosis. AIM-1 kinase has been reported to regulate late anaphase and cytokinesis. We have previously shown that AIM-1 mRNA is down-regulated upon Mpl ligand treatment of the a megakaryocytic cell line. Here, in order to examine the relevance of this kinase to polyploidization, tissue specific over-expression of AIM-1 in megakaryocytes in transgenic mice has been attempted. Transgenic AIM-1 mRNA was highly abundant in dipoidy as well as in high ploidy megakaryocytes, while AIM-1 protein was detected mainly at early stage of megakaryocyte differentiation, suggesting its regulation at protein level. This was accompanied by an increase in megakaryocyte number and proliferation potential, with no apparent impact on platelet number. Noted was also frequent neonatal death, as well as decreased megakarycyte ploidy level in the surviving transgenic mice. Our results indicated that AIM-1 plays an important role in megakaryocyte proliferation and polyploidization. In addition, our study suggested that AIM-1 level in megakaryocytes is regulated at both message and protein levels.

O-16

MAPPING OF SOMU1 AND M1 EPITOPES ON THE MUC5AC APOMUCIN, AN EARLY MARKER OF PANCREAS AND COLON CARCINOGENESIS

Jacques Bara, PhD, Séverine Nollet, PhD, Marie Elisabeth Forgue-Lafitte, PhD, Yoshio Okada, MD, PhD, Fabienne Escande, MD, Marie-Pierre Buisine, MD, PhD, Paul Kirkham, MD, PhD
U-482-INSERM, Hôpital S-Antoine, Paris; Okayama Prefectural University, Okayama, Japan;
U-377 INSERM, Place de Verdun, Lille - France; Novartis, Horsham, U.K.

The gastric M1 mucin, encoded by the MUC5AC gene, has been characterised by 11 anti-M1 monoclonal antibodies (MAbs). This mucin is an early marker of pancreatic and colon carcinogenesis. It is used to aid the diagnosis of mucinous pancreas cystadenomas, a precancerous lesion. Five anti-M1 MAbs (19M1, 21M1, 463M, 589M and 62M1) immunoreacted with the fragment of apomucin encoded the 3'end of MUC5AC gene and the epitopes have been mapped (Nollet et al., Int. J. Cancer 2002, 99: 336-343). In this study, we mapped 4 other epitopes by transfection of COS-7 cells with pSecTag2 B vectors containing different fragments of MUC5AC cDNA. Three gastric M1 epitopes: M1-a (MAb 1-13M1), M1-b (MAb 2-11M1), M1-d (MAb 9-13M1) and the SOMU1 epitope (Sotomozo et al., J Immunol. Methods 1996; 192:87-96) have been located in the N-terminal region of the MUC5AC apomucin: M1-a epitope is associated with the cys2 and cys4 domains, SOMU1 epitope with the cys5 domain, M1-b and M1-d epitopes with the globular D1/D2 and D3 domains, respectively. The three anti-M1 MAbs and the SOMU1 MAb stained the same goblet cells in serial sections of colon adenomas and mucosae adjacent to colon adenocarcinomas. The three remaining anti-M1 MAbs (2-12M1, 58M1 and 45M1) did not immunoreact with the products of the MUC5AC cDNA fragments we studied until now. The complete mapping of the M1 epitopes on the MUC5AC gene product will better characterise the tools required to improve the IRMA or ELISA measurement of M1/MUC5AC mucin in biological fluids.

O-17

THE CA125 GENE: THE REST OF THE STORY

Timothy J. O'Brien, PhD, John B. Beard, B.S., Lowell J. Underwood, PhD, Kazushi Shigemasa, MD, University of Arkansas for Medical Sciences, Arkansas; Hiroshima University Medical School, Hiroshima, Japan

At ISOBM in Barcelona, 2001, we described a CA125 structure which encompassed more than 11,000 amino acids and which was comprised of a carboxy terminus anchor region, a dominant repeat region and a relatively short (1637 amino acids) predominantly O-glycosylated amino terminal domain. This structure satisfied many of the known features of the CA125 molecule viz. a cytoplasmic tail capable of phosphorylation, a transmembrane domain, a potential extracellular cleavage site close to the plasma membrane, more than 60 repeat sequences of unique structure which individually are capable of binding the known classes of CA125 antibodies including M11 and OC125, and an amino terminal domain which could account for the known abundance of O-glycosylation in the CA125 molecule. Since our initial discoveries, we have continued to characterize adjacent genomic areas on chromosome 19 which we describe as the HLGP (hypothetical luminal glycoprotein) region. We now have evidence that an extensive nucleotide coding sequence (HLGP) is contiguous to and part of the 5' sequence of the CA125 molecule. We will present new data and sequencing of a significantly extended glycosylated amino terminal domain which supports a new amino acid composition for CA125 of 22,151, compared to our previously described composition of 11,720 amino acids. This gives CA125 a potential protein molecular weight of approximately 2.5 million daltons and the natural glycosylated form of at least 5 million daltons. This newly described CA125 moiety is consistent with the extraordinarily large molecular weight described by the ISOBM CA125 Workshop for CA125 found in peritoneal fluid or cervical mucous.

O-18

MEASUREMENT OF PROSTATE SPECIFIC ANTIGEN (PSA) AND HUMAN GLANDULAR KALLIKREIN (HK2) FROM BENIGN AND MALIGNANT PROSTATE TISSUE

Ville Väisänen, MSc, Pauliina Helo, Kalle A. Alanen, MD, Martti M.J. Nurmi, MD, Kim Pettersson, PhD
Department of Biotechnology, University of Turku, Department of Pathology, University Hospital Turku, Department of Urology, University Hospital Turku, Finland

PSA and hK2 levels in the bloodstream are elevated in patients with prostate cancer compared to healthy subjects. However, despite the numerous investigations made, it remains disputable whether the protein amounts are altered at a cellular level. It has become almost common knowledge, that PSA expression is lowered as cancer progresses, but opposing results have also been reported. Sample stability may have a profound effect on these results and could, at least in part, explain the discrepancies. The objective of this study was to extract and measure PSA and hK2 from cancerous and non-cancerous prostatic tissue, giving special consideration to sample stability.

Tissue samples were obtained from radical prostatectomies performed at the University Hospital of Turku. Immediately after removal of the prostate, core needle biopsy samples were taken into buffer containing protease inhibitors. All samples were frozen within one hour of removal of the prostate from the patient. Proteins were extracted with 1% Triton X-100 detergent and measured with in-house immunoassays specific for Total- and Free-PSA, Intact PSA and hK2. PSA and hK2 stability was monitored over time and repeated freeze/thaw cycles.

More than 90% of measured PSA was found to be in free uncomplexed form. Unlike in many previous studies, we could not observe any decrease of PSA content in cancerous tissue compared to non-cancerous controls. However, the amount of hK2 was significantly higher in cancerous than in non-cancerous tissue.

We report a method of tissue collection and extraction, which yields stable protein samples for immunometric measurements. We have measured the PSA and hK2 content of cancerous and non-cancerous tissue areas. Unlike previously reported by others, we could not observe a decrease of PSA in cancerous tissue. We did however see an increase in hK2, which could suggest a more important role of this protein as a tissue marker.

O-19

HIGH TELOMERASE EXPRESSION IN BARRETT'S ESOPHAGUS WITHOUT DYSPLASIA PREDICTS PROGRESSION TO ESOPHAGEAL ADENOCARCINOMA

Tarun Mullick, MD, Jason E. Tasch, PhD, Adrian H. Ormsby, MD, Paul Yeaton, MD, John Goldblum, MD, Robert E. Petras, MD, Terry L. Gramlich, MD, John Cowell, PhD, Gary W. Falk, MD, Joel E. Richter, MD
University of Virginia, Charlottesville, VA; Cleveland Clinic Foundation, Cleveland, OH; Henry Ford Institute, Detroit, MI; Rosewell Park Cancer Institute, Buffalo, NY

Background: Telomerase is a reverse transcriptase enzyme whose upregulation in cancer confers immortality. Previous work by our group in esophagectomy specimens showed telomerase upregulation in areas of intestinal metaplasia without dysplasia adjacent to cancer (Am J Gastro 2001;96:A75).**AIMS:**To determine if positive telomerase expression in Barrett's esophagus patients could predict the subsequent development of esophageal adenocarcinoma. **Methods:**16 patients with long-segment Barrett's esophagus (> 3 cm) with a diagnosis of low-grade dysplasia were followed in an endoscopic surveillance program. 7 patients eventually progressed to esophageal adenocarcinoma, while 9 patients did not over a mean of 9.3 years of follow-up. Biopsies of intestinal metaplasia without dysplasia and subsequent biopsies of low-grade dysplasia were examined with telomerase enzyme immunostaining and were assessed by 4 blinded GI pathologists(consensus was 3/4 agreeing). Positive nuclear telomerase enzyme expression in biopsies with intestinal metaplasia without dysplasia was compared between the patients who progressed to cancer and those who did not to determine if positive telomerase enzyme expression in intestinal metaplasia without dysplasia predicted the subsequent development of esophageal adenocarcinoma. Concurrently, p53, cyclin D1, and bcl-2 were assayed by immunohistochemistry. **Results:** Of the 7 progressors to cancer, telomerase was positive in all 7, while being negative in all 9 non-progressors. p53 and bcl-2 were not positive in any patient, while cyclin d1 was positive in 6/7 progressors and 7/9 non-progressors. Telomerase expression was upregulated in endoscopic surveillance biopsies of intestinal metaplasia without dysplasia between 0 and 8 cm away from the eventual cancer and was detected 2.6(range 0.5 to 10 years) before the onset of cancer.Positive telomerase enzyme expression's ability to predict progression to cancer in intestinal metaplasia was statistically significant ($p < 0.001$). Other potential biomarkers as shown above did not approach this sensitivity and specificity. **Conclusion:**1) Positive telomerase enzyme expression present in intestinal metaplasia without dysplasia predicted all those patients who progressed to develop esophageal adenocarcinoma. p53, cyclin D1,and bcl-2 were not as sensitive or specific.2) Positive telomerase enzyme expression precedes histological development of dysplasia. This is the first biomarker in the Barrett's-adenocarcinoma sequence to predict cancer at the level of intestinal metaplasia without dysplasia, a major breakthrough. 3) Telomerase merits further evaluation as a biomarker of stratification of Barrett's esophagus patients in endoscopic surveillance programs.

O-20

DEVELOPMENT OF IMMUNOASSAYS FOR MEASUREMENT OF DIFFERENT MOLECULAR FORMS OF HUMAN GLANDULAR KALLIKREIN 2 (HK2)

Ville Väisänen, MSc, Susann Eriksson, MSc, Kaisa Ivaska, MSc, Hans Lilja, MD, PhD, Kim Pettersson, PhD
Department of Biotechnology, University of Turku, Finland, Department of Clinical Chemistry, Lund University, Malmö, Sweden

HK2 is a close homologue to PSA and can be predominantly found in the prostate. It has been shown to be a prostate cancer (PC) marker of independent value. Immunoassays for detection of hK2 must be very sensitive, since concentrations of serum hK2 are very low. HK2 alone or in combination with forms of PSA enables an improved detection of PC of higher grade and stage. The present study aimed to develop immunoassays with the required sensitivity for both free and complexed forms of hK2.

hK2, similarly to PSA; can exist in several different molecular forms (complexed, free, pro-form, internally nicked). Three monoclonal antibodies (6H10, 7D7, 11B6) raised against hK2 have shown variable recognition of these different molecular forms of hK2. The Mabs were used either as capture or tracer Mabs to construct two-site immunoassays with altered specificities to different molecular forms of hK2. This kind of assays would enable investigations of the possible diagnostic or prognostic role of different molecular forms of hK2 in PC.

The developed assays have been tested for their ability to measure different forms of hK2 (pro-form, mature and nicked hK2) as well as hK2-complexes. Clinically non-characterised serum samples were used for a first evaluation of the assays. The cross-reactivities of the Mabs for hK2 in complex with ACT, PCI, PAI-1 and AT were as follows; 6H10: 96, 65, 73 and 41%; 11B6: 2, 31, 26 and 35% and 7D7: 7, 4, 5 and 24% respectively. All of the developed assays had a detection limit of about 4 ng/L, but they showed a differing recognition pattern for different recombinant forms of hK2. They also gave significantly different values for hK2 measured from serum samples. Free hK2 comprises about 95% of the total amount of hK2 found in serum.

Highly sensitive and specific assays for hK2 with distinct specificity profiles towards different molecular forms of hK2 were established. These assays will be used for defining the possible role of different forms of hK2 in PC.

O-21

PROTEOMIC ANALYSIS OF ARSENIC-INDUCED CELL TRANSFORMATION

Andy T. Lau, PhD, Qing-Yu He, PhD, Muyao Li, MD, Hsiang-fu Kung, PhD, Chi-Ming Che, PhD, Jen-Fu Chiu, PhD
Institute of Molecular Biology, Department of Chemistry, University of Hong Kong, Hong Kong; Department of Medicine, University of Vermont, Burlington, VT

Recent epidemiological studies and clinical observations have associated arsenics with an increased risk of human cancer, including urinary bladder, liver, kidney, skin, lung nasal cavity, prostate, and other internal sites. Despite a wealth of epidemiologic and clinic data, the mechanisms by which arsenite cause cancers are still unknown. To gain insight into the biological effects of arsenic and to identify gene activity relevant to its cell transformation, the changes of protein expression profiles during cell transformation were analyzed by proteomic technology.

Since arsenic acts as a tumor promoter, we used carcinogen, B[a]P, as a tumor initiator to mutate cellular DNA. LEC cells were treated with 100 nm B[a]P for 24 hr and then divided into two groups. Each treatment contains three plates. The first group of culture continued to grow under a regular culture medium. The second group of cultures grew in a regular medium, plus 1.5 mM soudium arsenic for 12 weeks. Cells were then plated in soft agar to see the effect of arsenite on cell transformation by determining anchorage independent growth. 483 colonies on soft agar were formed by cells treated with 100 nm B[a]P for 24 hr and 1.5 mM arsenite for 12 weeks. 35 colonies were identified from cells that treated with B[a]P alone. No colony was formed in both control cells and cells only treated with As.

We then analyzed the proteomic response to arsenite to identify protein expression by Protein Chips. These ProteinChips were coated with either metal compound (Cu-affinity ProteinChip), Strong anion exchanger (SAX ProteinChip), or weak cation exchanger (WCX ProteinChip), respectively. Most of protein peaks in cell extracts of all samples, including control, B[a]P-treated, and B[a]P+As-treated cells are identical. However, SELDI-TOF analysis revealed several dramatic different protein peaks appeared in LEC cells after transformed by long-term treatment with low level of arsenic (1.5 mM for 12 weeks). Analysis of cellular protein profiles from control and experimental LEC cells, Sax chip revealed that one prominent protein peak was preferentially expressed in control cells. Interestingly, using SAX chip, we were able to detect several protein peaks that increased their expression in LEC cells treated only with B[a]P. Identification and characterization of these protein may reveal the molecular basis of As-induced cell proliferation and provide insight into the mechanisms by which arsenic-induced carciongenesis.

O-22

TOPICAL CHEMOPREVENTION OF ORAL CANCER WITH POLYMER-DELIVERED RETINOIC ACID

Zhi Wang, MD, Raju Polavaram, MD, Cesar F. Fuentes, MD, Stanley M. Shapshay, MD
Department of Otolaryngology, Boston University School of Medicine, Boston, MA

Objective: Oral cancer is a common malignancy. Chemoprevention is a promising therapy but its extensive application is hampered by systemic toxicity. Topical chemoprevention provides an attractive strategy in an attempt to reduce such side-effect. This study is based on a hypothesis that use of mucosal adherent film (MAF), as a vehicle to topically deliver retinoic acid (RA), can significantly improve efficacy with current methods in topical chemoprevention of oral cancer. **Methods:** Cheek pouch of hamster was painted with DMBA for 5 weeks to result in premalignant lesions on buccal mucosa. 36 hamsters were then divided into 3 groups, 12 of each: (1) control: no treatment; (2) systemic medication: 5.0 mg RA/kg/day, IP; and (3) topical MAF: topical MAF patch (containing 2.25 mg RA/cm2) placed on the lesion, once daily. The treatment was continued for 40 days, and the tumor growth was measured to evaluate the treatment efficacy. MAF retention time on mucosa and local tissue tolerance to MAF were also observed in additional 17 hamsters. **Results:** Statistically, there was significant difference in the tumor growth between the control and MAF group ($p < 0.0001$). The topical MAF patch produced comparable efficacy to that treated with the systemic RA ($p > 0.1$). MAF could remain on applied site at least for 5 hours, and was well tolerated by mucosa. **Discussions:** Current mainstay of topical chemoprevention of oral cancer consists of brief solution painting. It is difficult to ensure the applied agent with adequate concentration and sufficient retention time on tissue due to excessive saliva flash and frequent oral activities. MAF made with water-soluble polymer has been successfully used in oral cavity for topically delivering analgesics, antibiotics or other medications. It provides improved efficacy during its extended retention on site for hours. However, none has used MAF technique to date for oral cancer prevention. **Conclusion:** This study has shown, for the first time, that MAF-delivered RA is effective for topical chemoprevention of oral cancer.

O-23

CYCLOOXYGENASE-2 EXPRESSION AS RELATED TO A GENETIC RISK MARKER OF ORAL CANCER

Bryne Magne, PhD, Sondresen Jan, DDS, Ristimaki Ari, MD, PhD, Reith Albrecht, MD, PhD, Sudbø Jon, MD, PhD
Department of Oral Biology, University of Oslo, Norway, Department of Pathology, University of Hensinki, Finland, Department of Pathology, Norwegian Radium Hospital, Oslo, Norway, Department of Oncology, Norwegian Radium Hospital, Oslo, Norway

Purpose, Patients and Methods: To see if individuals at considerably increased risk of oral cancer are candidates for treatment with selective cyclooxygenase-2 inhibitors (coxibs), levels of cyclooxygenase-2 expression in healthy, premalignant and cancerous oral mucosa were compared to the occurrence of a genetic risk marker of oral cancer. Cyclooxygenase-2 gene product was detected immunohistochemically in 30 healthy persons, in 22 patients with dysplastic lesions without previous or concomitant carcinomas, and in 29 patients with oral carcinomas. Cyclooxygenase-2 expression was compared to DNA content as a genetic risk marker of oral cancer. Follow-up data were available for all patients with premalignant and malignant lesions. **Results:** Cyclooxygenase-2 expression was found in 1 case of healthy oral mucosa (3 percent). All specimens from healthy mucosa had a normal DNA content. Of 22 patients with dysplastic lesions, 9 (41 percent) expressed cyclooxygenase-2, of which all had aberrant (aneuploid) DNA content. A carcinoma developed in 6 of 7 patients with cyclooxygenase-2 expressing lesions with aberrant DNA content that were followed for 5 years or more (85 percent; P=0.02). None of the patients with diploid lesions developed a carcinoma during follow up. In 29 patients with oral carcinomas, cyclooxygenase-2 expression was observed in 26 (88 percent), and aneuploidy was observed in 25 cases (94 percent, P = 0.04). **Conclusion:** Cyclooxygenase-2 was up-regulated from healthy to premalignant to cancerous oral mucosa. In patients with premalignancies, cyclooxygenase-2 was exclusively expressed in a subgroup identified to be at considerably increased risk of cancer by an aberrant DNA content. These findings emphasize the need to determine whether coxibs can reduce the risk of oral cancer in patients with high-risk precancerous lesions.

O-24

POLYCLONAL ANTIBODY LIBRARIES FOR CANCER TREATMENT

Jacqueline Sharon, PhD, Brent R. Williams, PhD, Liyan Chen, MD, Sanda Teodorescu-Frumosu, MD
Department of Pathology, Boston University School of Medicine, Boston, MA

Preliminary studies have shown that serum or purified antibodies from mice immunized with the human colon cancer cell line SW480 caused significant growth retardation or complete regression of established SW480 tumor xenografts in immunodeficient nude mice. To capitalize and improve on this multi-thronged approach to cancer therapy, we are developing anti-colorectal cancer polyclonal antibody libraries. These are standardized mixtures of anti-colorectal cancer antibodies, for which the genes are available and therefore the antibodies can be perpetuated, amplified, and modified as desired; for example to create chimeric antibodies with human constant regions or all-human antibodies. An anti-cancer polyclonal antibody library will contain both cancer-specific and cross-reactive antibodies but is designed to recognize the antigenic profile of cancer cells over the antigenic profiles of normal cells, with a high signal-to-noise ratio. Following our system for polyclonal antibody library generation, we have selected Fab phage display libraries reactive with human colorectal cancer cell lines and depleted of reactivity to human blood cells. These libraries were shown to contain 50-90% antigen-reactive clones despite remaining diverse. A prototypic polyclonal antibody library, comprising full-length IgG antibodies, was generated by mass transfer of VL-VH region gene pairs from a selected anti-colorectal cancer Fab phage display library to a mammalian expression vector followed by transfection of the resulting vector library into myeloma cells. Experiments in progress will compare the anti-tumor efficacy of the polyclonal antibody library with that of the clinically-used anti-colorectal cancer monoclonal antibody 17-1A and other monoclonal and oligoclonal antibodies.

O-25

ATTENUATED SALMONELLA TYPHIMURIUM PREVENTS THE ESTABLISHMENT OF HEPATIC COLORECTAL METASTASES AND IMPROVES SURVIVAL IN A MURINE MODEL

Leland J. Soto III, MD, Brent S. Sorenson, BS, Adam S. Kim, BS, Brad A. Feltis, MD, Arnold S. Leonard, MD, PhD, Daniel A. Saltzman, MD, PhD
University of Minnesota, Minneapolis, MN

Purpose: We previously reported that attenuated Salmonella typhimurium that contains the human gene for interleukin-2 (Salmonella-pIL2) is effective in the treatment of unresectable hepatic metastases. This study defines the optimal timing of oral Salmonella to prevent hepatic metastases, quantifies the hepatic lymphocyte response and survival benefit.
Methods: Attenuated S. typhimurium (no gene), Salmonella-pIL2 or saline was given orally to mice. Eight days later, a model of unresectable hepatic metastases was established. Animals were randomized to cyclooxygenase-2 inhibition (COX-2i) post-operatively to achieve six groups (n=18 each). Liver tumors were enumerated on post-operative day 14. Hepatic natural killer (NK), CD8+ and CD4+ cells were evaluated by flow cytometry. Survival study mimicked above (n=13-16 each). Animals surviving 90 days were sacrificed.
Results: Ten-fold reductions in tumor number were seen in Salmonella treated groups compared to controls (9.2 and 5.9 vs 77.7; Fisher's exact test, p<0.0001). COX-2i provided a smaller reduction in tumor number (57; p=0.03) but no synergy with Salmonella. Treatment with Salmonella resulted in a greater than two-fold increase in hepatic NK populations (14.3% and 13.6% vs 5.8%; p<0.0001). Similarly, CD8+ lymphocytes were elevated in Salmonella groups (12% and 11.1% vs 7.2%; p<0.01). A smaller rise in CD4+ T-cells was noted in Salmonella groups. COX-2i alone did not change lymphocyte populations. Survival advantages were seen in Salmonella groups (mean 56 days vs 21 days; p<0.04 Breslow-Wilcoxon). Accordingly, 30-33% of Salmonella treated animals survived 90 days, all of which were devoid of hepatic tumor. COX-2i did not change survival.
Conclusion: Orally dosed attenuated Salmonella typhimurium represents a novel form of immunotherapy to prevent the establishment of hepatic metastases. The anti-tumor effect is associated with elevated hepatic NK, CD8+ lymphocytes.

O-26

IMPORTANCE OF DIAGNOSTIC LEVEL AS THE GOLD STANDARD FOR EVALUATION OF ALPHA-FETOPROTEIN AND ITS GLYCOFORMS AS MARKERS OF HEPATOCELLULAR CARCINOMA

Kazuhisa Taketa, MD
Department of Internal Medicine, Ibara City Hospital, Ibara, Japan

Serum level of alpha-fetoprotein (AFP) has been widely used as a marker of hepatocellular carcinoma (HCC). However, AFP level also increases in benign chronic liver diseases (CLD), chronic hepatitis and cirrhosis, which are the underlying conditions of HCC evolution. As a result of advances in imaging techniques, AFP levels of HCC became lower and widely overlapping with those of CLD. Thus, serum AFP determination was less useful for diagnosis of early HCC, although small rises in AFP in CLD were shown to be significant predictor of future evolution of HCC. On the other hand, AFP glycoforms, particularly AFP-L3 and AFP-P4, were more specific markers of HCC and could be used as diagnostic markers. However, the sensitivity of AFP-L3 and AFP-P4 was low in well-differentiated HCC or HCC with tumor diameters less than 2 cm. Decreasing cutoff levels did not increase the specificity appreciably and it rather caused decrease in specificity. Combined evaluation of AFP-L3 and AFP-P4 increased sensitivity without decreasing specificity. These AFP glycoforms were useful markers to predict prognosis or recurrence after therapeutic intervention. On the contrary, the specificity of AFP glycoforms were low when HCC was not ruled out extensively by imaging in diagnosis of CLD. Accordingly, the evaluation of HCC markers largely depends on the diagnostic level of HCC as the gold standard.

O-27

SENSITIVE AND SPECIFIC ENZYMATIC ASSAY FOR THE DETERMINATION OF PRECURSOR FORMS OF PROSTATE-SPECIFIC ANTIGEN AFTER ACTIVATION STEP

Pauliina M Niemela, MSc, Janita Lövgren, PhD, Matti Karp, PhD, Hans Lilja, MD, PhD, Kim Pettersson, PhD
University of Turku, Turku, Finland; Lund University, Lund, Sweden

Background: Precursor forms of PSA (proPSA) have been shown to be a portion of free PSA in blood of patients with prostatic disorders. However, the diagnostic potential of proPSA forms has not been established due to lack of sensitive methods to measure these forms. We have developed a specific and sensitive method for the measurement of active PSA and used it to measure proPSA forms of 4 amino acids or longer by applying an activation step that converts inactive proPSA to active PSA.

Methods: Synthetic peptide KGISSQY that possesses a PSA-specific cleavage site was used for the detection of active PSA. To ascertain the specificity of the assay, an anti-PSA Mab was used to capture known forms of PSA. Inactive proPSA was converted to active, mature PSA by human glandular kallikrein 2.

Results: The detection limit of the optimized assay was 0.5 µg/L. In blood samples from patients, the activation step substantially increased the concentration of active PSA, thus showing the presence of proPSA in the samples. ProPSA was 0-79% (median=45%) of the amount of free PSA in 15 samples with total PSA concentrations 5.3-423 µg/L. In samples obtained from three benign prostatic hyperplasia (BPH) patients after transurethal resection of the prostate (TUR-P), no significant increase of activity was detected after the activation step, thus showing that proPSA was not a portion of free PSA in blood of BPH patients.

Conclusions: Pro-forms are a considerable fraction of free PSA in blood of patients with increased total PSA. The approach described can be used to study the role and concentrations of active PSA and proPSA in different body fluids and tissue extracts. Also, the diagnostic value of proPSA in benign and prostate cancer patients remains to be clarified.

O-28

SERUM S-100B: A PROGNOSTIC MARKER IN MALIGNANT MELANOMA

Lars-Olof Hansson, MD, PhD, Eva Djureen Mårtenson, MD, Bo Nilsson, Johan Hansson, MD, PhD, Ulrik Ringborg, MD
Department of Oncology, Clinical Chemistry and Cancer Epidemiology, Karolinska Hospital, Stockholm, Sweden

Background: In melanoma patients the prognosis has been steadily increased during the last decades. However, despite these advances 20 to 25 % of melanoma patients will develop loco-regional and/or distant metastasis and the majority of them consequently die. Serum levels of S-100B are correlated to clinical stage and strongly associated to overall survival especially in stage III and IV patients.

Objectives: To investigate whether S-100B in serum is a prognostic marker in follow-up of patients with malignant melanoma. S-100B protein levels in serum were also measured in 412 healthy adult subjects to establish a reference interval.

The study: S-100B in serum was measured, initially, in 1047 consecutive patients with histologically proven cutaneous malignant melanoma and repetitively during follow up in 69 patients with progressive disease. The median follow-up time of the patients was about 5 years. S-100B was measured using a chemoluminometric (Sangtec 100, Sangtec Medical, Bromma, Sweden).

Summary of results: The geometric mean value in the healthy reference group was 0.02 mg/l and 95% of the individuals had values £ 0.10 mg/l. No sex-related differences were found. Results will also be shown for S-100 B in different benign and malignant diseases. The mean serum concentration of S-100B protein was significantly related to clinical stage. In the multivariate analysis S-100B protein level in serum was the strongest independent prognostic factor in advanced stages ($p<0.001$; RH=2.08) followed by clinical stage ($p=0.005$; RH=1.92). S-100 B had a strong predictive value with respect to progression ($p<0.001$) in the 69 patients with progressive disease.

O-29

A SINGLE-CHAIN ANTIBODY SPECIFIC FOR MECONIUM CEA (NCA-2): DEVELOPMENT, CHARACTERIZATION AND USE IN IMMUNOASSAY

Elisabeth Paus, PhD, Hilde Almåsbak, Ole P. Børmer, MD, PhD, Johan Bjerner, MD, David J. Warren, MD
The Norwegian Radium Hospital, Oslo, Norway

Aim: Carcinoembryonic antigen (CEA) is a member of the immunglobulin gene superfamily. In meconium a variant of CEA is predominant, characterized by lack of the C-terminal epitopes, and denominated meconium CEA or NCA-2. It has been shown that this molecular variant may be present also in serum from adult cancer patients, but no NCA-2 specific assay is available, and the possible clinical significance is largely unknown. We have used phage-display technology to produce single-chain variable antibody fragments (scFv) suitable for a NCA-2 specific assay, and compared the NCA-2 results with CEA values in patient sera. **Methods:** Single chain Fv antibody fragments were selected from a phage display library made from splenic mRNA of an immunized mouse. NCA-2 purified from meconium was used as the antigen. Expression was performed in E.coli, and biosensor technology was used to map and select a high affinity scFv. The antibody fragment was labeled with Eu-chelate and applied as tracer antibody in a two-site assay for NCA-2. For comparison we used our routine assay for CEA, which measures CEA and NCA-2 equivalently, and a CEA-specific assay based on the T84.66 antibody (C.Wagener & J. Shively). **Results:** After two rounds of panning on solid phase coated with NCA-2, several clones were selected and cloned into an E.coli expression vector. From the BiaCore studies a scFv with low koff and a Kd of 10-10 mol/l was selected for Eu-labelling, and an immunofluorometric assay with a sensitivity of 0.2 ng/ml was established. The assay detects a protein in serum with a molecular weight like NCA-2, significantly lower than CEA. The difference between serum values measured with the two CEA assays corresponded to the values determined with the NCA-2 assay. **Conclusion:** An immunoassay based on a scFv antibody with high affinity for NCA-2 measures only the non-specific cross-reacting antigen-2 with no or minor cross-reaction to CEA.

O-30

PROHIBITIN REQUIRES BRG-1 AND BRM FOR THE REPRESSION OF E2F AND CELL GROWTH

Sheng Wang, PhD, Baohua Zhang, MD, Douglas V. Faller, MD, PhD
Cancer Research Center, Boston University School of Medicine, Boston, MA

The E2F transcription factors play major role in controlling mammalian cell cycle progression. Expression of many genes necessary for S-phase progression requires E2F. E2F is important down stream target of Rb tumor suppressor. Viral onco-proteins, like SV40Tag can affect the ability of Rb to repress E2F. We recently reported that a potential tumor suppressor, prohibitin, regulates E2F function, and this activity correlates with its growth suppressive function. There are important differences between Rb and Prohibitin. Our deletion analysis identified that the highly conserved marked box region of E2F is targeted by prohibitin, unlike Rb, which binds to the E2F transcriptional domain. Furthermore, our study revealed differential regulation of the Rb- and prohibitin-mediated E2F repression by upstream signals.

Recent evidence demonstrated the involvement of members of SWI/SNF family in the Rb-mediated repression of E2F. Results from our immuno-precipitation/western blot analysis indicate that prohibitin interact with Brg-1 and Brm in vivo. Expression of a dominant negative Brg-1 or Brm releases prohibitin-mediated repression of E2F and relieves prohibitin-mediated growth suppression. Chromosome immuno-precipitation assays (CHIP) confirmed that prohibitin recruits Brg-1 and Brm to repress both transfected as well as natural E2F responsive promoters. A viral onco-protein, SV40Tag, can reverse prohibitin-mediated suppression of E2F, and targets prohibitin through interruption of the association between prohibitin and Brg-1/Brm without affecting the prohibitin and E2F interaction. This result is in distinct contrast to the effect of SV40Tag on Rb-mediated gene suppression, wherein Rb itself is dissociated from the promoter by the viral onco-protein. This result thus defines a novel type of functional interaction for SV40Tag with transcriptional regulators, as well as demonstrating a new level of regulation in Brg-1/Brm co-repressor/transcription complex interactions.

O-31

CARCINOEMBRYONIC ANTIGEN RECEPTOR EXPRESSION AND SIGNALING IN KUPFFER CELLS

Peter Thomas, PhD, Regis Zimmer, PhD,DVM, Gina Stolper, MD, Olga V Bajenova, PhD
Boston University School of Medicine, Boston, MA

Elevated amounts of carcinoembryonic antigen (CEA) in the blood is associated with the development of hepatic metastases from colorectal cancers. Clearance of circulating CEA occurs through the binding to a surface receptor on liver macrophages (Kupffer cells). The rat Kupffer cell CEA receptor (CEAR) has been identified as one of two known isoforms of heterogeneous nuclear RNA binding protein M4 (hnRNP M4). This isoform has a 29 amino-acid deletion between RNA-binding domain 1 and 2 close to the N-terminus. We also have evidence for at least two other splicing forms in macrophage cell lines. Binding of CEA to its receptor results in production of cytokines that influence the tumors ability to implant and grow in the liver. In Kupffer cells CEA binding causes the activation of a number of transcription factors including NfkB and AP-1 which are known to be involved in the synthesis of cytokines. Transfection of p388D1 macrophages with CEAR cDNA also resulted in CEA binding and cytokine production. We have produced 3 polyclonal anti-CEAR antibodies. Two of them to the N-terminal part of CEAR can specifically recognize the CEAR and the full length hnRNP M4, and the third antibody to the C-terminus is specific to both isoforms.. Using these antibodies we showed by FACS analyses that the CEA receptor is expressed on the surface of Kupffer cells and CEAR transfected p388D1 macrophages. Immunoprecipitation with antibody to the CEAR C-terminal domain showed that CEAR protein expression is up-regulated in Kupffer cells in response to CEA and that binding initiates formation of a protein complex that includes beta-actin. These results suggest that CEA initiates a complex signaling cascade in Kupffer cells that is distinct from that of other activators such as LPS. The role of the two receptor isoforms is being elucidated in Kupffer and other cells. There is evidence that these proteins can also bind CEA in cancer cells but not as a surface receptor. This has implications in tumor cell growth and the development of metastasis.

O-32

DECREASED EGFR IN CANCER SERA

Marilee Burrell, BS, Leticia D. Morris, BS, Walter P. Carney, PhD, Peter J. Hamer, MA
Oncogene Science/Bayer Diagnostics, Cambridge, MA

Transmembrane growth factor receptors are important in many aspects of signal transduction. The uncontrolled signaling through some receptors has been implicated in the process of oncogenesis. We have studied the expression of the ErbB family of growth factor receptors, specifically the epidermal growth factor receptor (EGFr or erbB-1). EGFr exists as a full-length transmembrane receptor with a molecular weight (MW) of 170 kDa, while the extracellular domain (ECD) has an MW of 110 kDa. We have developed a commercially available microtiter ELISA for the detection and quantitation of the ECD of EGFr in human serum samples. Initial work focused on obtaining a reliable range for the level of EGFr ECD in normal individuals. To that end we analyzed over 200 normal serum samples using the Oncogene Science EGFr Microtiter ELISA. The samples were divided between males and females. Results showed that the mean level of EGFr ECD in normal males was 62 ng/mL and in normal females was 61 ng/mL. The range of normal values, as determined by the mean value +/- two standard deviations (SD) was 45 - 78 ng/mL of EGFr ECD. We then analyzed serum samples from a number of cancer patients, including breast, bladder, colon, lung, ovarian and prostate. Surprisingly, results showed that in all cancer types tested, a large percentage of the samples had EGFr ECD levels that were decreased below the normal range. In the bladder cancers 56% of the samples had decreased values, 46% of the colon cancers had decreased EGFr ECD and 44% of the prostate cancers had decreased EGFr ECD. In the ovarian cancer serum samples, results showed that as the cancer stage increased there were a larger percentage of samples with decreased EGFr ECD. Specifically, in the stage I ovarian cancers 29% of the samples had decreased EGFr ECD, while in the stage IV ovarian cancer sera 78% of the samples had a decreased EGFr ECD. There are several reasons why the EGFr ECD levels may be decreased in cancer patient sera. It may be that there is the elaboration of anti-EGFr antibodies which complex with the EGFr ECD and the antigen-antibody complex is then cleared from the circulation. Alternatively, there could be an increase in EGFr ligands, which could bind the full-length transmembrane EGFr and cause downregulation of EGFr. Evaluation of serum levels of EGFr ECD may prove useful in the application of EGFr specific therapies that are currently under development.

O-33

THE "REMAINING FOLLICLE HYPOTHESIS" - A NEW HYPOTHESIS OF THE ETIOLOGY AND PATHOGENESIS OF OVARIAN CANCER

Wolfram H. Jaeger, MD, PhD
Department GynOncol University of Erlangen, Germany

In previous studies we could demonstrate in a rat model that continuous stimulation of the ovary by gonadotropins causes cancer in these ovaries. We further found that cysts of human ovarian cancer contain LH and FSH, while these gonadotropins were never found in benign cysts. Furthermore only ovarian cancer cysts sometimes contain estrogen and hCG. Ovarian cancer cells in culture are able to produce estrogens and hcG, but not LH and FSH. We furthermore measured a typical spectrum of different proteins in these cysts which led us to conclude that after diffusion of LH and FSH in these cancer cysts these egonadotropins don´t do anything strange, but simply induce their physiological effects - steroid hormone production. In the postmenopausal ovary this could probably not be done by the epithelium or the stroma, but by the remaining primordial follicles after menopause and their surrounding granulosa and theca cells. The continuous high gonadotropins can probably not induce the remaining primordial follicles deep in the stroma to produce a follicle (too much physical pressure by the surrounding connective tissue), but remaining follicles close to the ovarian surface. They than start folliculargenesis by building up a cyst ("follicle") and produce and secret estrogens and LDH among others. At a special time - caused by some unknown events - these cells furthermore induce the mechanisms which would usually be neccessary for implantation of the blastocyst: they induce angiogenesis and produce hCG. As long as the cysts do not rupture this process will restrict to the ovary, however, when the cysts rupture, the cells can "implant" on the peritoneal surface and lead to the typical picture of advanced ovarian cancer.

One could therefore hypothesize that the continuous stimulation of remaining primordial follicles - not at the surface but close to the surface of the ovary - is the critical event in the etiology of ovarian cancer. The "pathogenesis" of the disease then follows the usual course of the events during follicular maturation and implantation. It sounds strange, but according to this hypoothesis "pathegenesis" is "physiology" at the wrong time!

(N.B. The "repeated rupture and repair" etiology of ovarian cancer proposed by Fathalla, can not be tested and is therefore not considered a hypothesis by the author, as well as the speculation that "high gonadotropins" must be involved in the causative events.)

O-34

THE DOMINANT NEGATIVE INHIBITOR OF INSULIN-LIKE GROWTH FACTOR-I RECEPTOR IS PROMISING STRATEGY FOR HUMAN COLON AND PANCREATIC CANCER CELLS

Yasushi Adachi, MD, PhD, Yongfen Min, MD, Hiroyuki Yamamoto, MD, PhD, Tadao Ishida, MD, PhD, Fumio Itoh, MD, PhD, Yasuo Kato, MD, PhD, Choon-Taek Lee, MD, PhD, Sorena Nadaf, Kohzoh Imai, MD, PhD, David P Carbone, MD, PhD
Sapporo Medical University, Sapporo, Japan; Vanderbilt University Medical Center, Nashville, TN

Continuous tumor growth depends on the altered regulation of the cell cycle that is in turn modulated by signals from growth factors and their receptors, including insulin-like growth factors (IGF) and IGF-I receptor (IGF-Ir). It has been reported that blockade of IGF-Ir by antisense or dominant negative plasmid transfection can suppress tumorigenicity and induce regression of established tumors. In order to study the mechanism of this effect and develop potential targeted therapeutics, we have constructed two truncated IGF-Irs (482 and 950 amino acid long, IGF-Ir/482st and IGF-Ir/950st, respectively) that function as dominant negative inhibitors (IGF-Ir/dn) which were cloned into recombinant adenoviruses. The effects of these adenoviruses were studied in human colon and pancreatic cancer cell lines. We assessed efficiency of IGF-Ir signaling blockade, the effect of IGF-Ir/dn on cell growth, steady-state, radiation, and chemotherapy induced apoptosis, and in vivo therapeutic efficacy in xenografts. The IGF-Ir/dn suppressed tumorigenicity of cancer cells both in vitro and in vivo and increased the amount of steady-state apoptosis in cancer cells. IGF-Ir/dn effectively blocked both IGF-I and IGF-II signaling through Akt-1 and IGF-Ir/482st showed a bystander effect. IGF-Ir/dn increased chemotherapy and radiation induced apoptosis in vitro and the combination therapy of chemotherapy and IGF-Ir/dn was very effective against established tumors in mice. Moreover, IGF-Ir/482st more effectively suppressed tumor growth than IGF-Ir/950st. These data suggest that IGF-Ir/dn, especially IGF-Ir/482st, may be a useful therapeutic strategy for colorectal and pancreatic cancers.

O-35

A PHASE I, DOSE-ESCALATING, PHARMACOKINETIC (PK) AND PHARMACODYNAMIC (PD) STUDY OF PTK787/ZK 222584 (PTK/ZK) IN PATIENTS WITH ADVANCED RENAL CELL OR PROSTATE CARCINOMAS

Daniel J. George, MD, Eric Jonasch, MD, William K. Oh, MD, Laura A. Hart, Parker Kathryn, PhD, Andrew Henry, Margaret Dugan, MD, Dirk Laurent, Philip W. Kantoff, MD, William G. Kaelin, MD
Dana-Farber Cancer Institute, Massachusetts General Hospital, Boston, MA; Novartis Pharmaceuticals, E. Hanover, NJ; Schering AG, Berlin, Germany

Vascular endothelial growth factor (VEGF) is a prominent pro-angiogenic growth factor produced by many solid tumor cell types, including prostate (CaP) and renal cell carcinomas (RCC), and represents a new therapeutic target. We performed a Phase I, dose-escalating study of PTK787/ZK 222584 (PTK/ZK), a potent and selective small molecule inhibitor of KDR and Flt-1 (VEGF receptors) that has demonstrated anti-tumor and anti-angiogenic activity in pre-clinical models (Cancer Res 60: 2178-2189, 2000 and Cancer Res 60: 4819-4824, 2000). The purpose of our investigation was to determine the safety and maximum tolerated dose of once daily, orally administered PTK/ZK in these patient populations as well as to determine the biologically active range for optimal Phase II and Phase III dosing. To date, 21 patients with metastatic RCC have been enrolled (17 evaluable), 6 with no prior therapy and 15 who had 1- 4 prior therapies. Three CaP patients (all evaluable) failing primary hormonal therapy were enrolled. Patients were evaluated for biologic response with dynamic, contrast-enhanced magnetic resonance imaging (DCE-MRI) and circulating biomarker measurements. Cohorts of 3 patients were treated at each dose level, which was expanded to six patients if a dose limiting toxicity (DLT) was observed. A total of five dose levels (300 - 1500 mg) have been completed to date and no MTD has been established. Single cases of grade III toxicity (headache, hypertension, nausea) have been observed at 1000 - 1500 mg dose levels. The most frequent adverse events include nausea, headache, fatigue, and dizziness. Based on safety data, pharmacokinetics, DCE-MRI findings and clinical responses in several other phase I studies, a biologically active dose range has been identified as >=1000 mg/day. We have treated 15 patients (age range 51-76; M:F 12:3) with progressive metastatic RCC (all with adenocarcinoma, clear cell histology) at doses of 1000-1500 mg/day (10 evaluable for response). All 10 were progression free at 2 months, with median progression-free survival of six months (range 4-11 months). Five of 10 patients are still on treatment (range of 6-11 months). Currently, an extended cohort of 25 RCC patients are being accrued at 1200 mg/day to better define this biologically active dose.

O-36

MOLECULAR GENETIC PROFILING OF INTERFERON RESPONSIVE RENAL CELL CARCINOMA

Louis S. Liou, MD, BA, Michelle Holko, Marek Skacel, MD, Joseph DiDonato, PhD, Bryan Williams, PhD, Andrew Novick, MD
Cleveland Clinic Foundation, Cleveland Heights, OH

Background and Objective: Interferon (IFN) has previously been the mainstay of immunotherapy in patients with metastatic renal cell carcinoma (RCC). Although the response rate is low there are rare cases of complete responses. The tumor prognostic molecular variables identifying the small subset of IFN sensitive RCC are still unknown. We investigate the genetic profile of a complete IFN responder and compare this to the profile of surgically excised IFN naïve patients.

Materials and Methods: We present a patient with metastatic RCC who had a complete response to IFN and subsequently underwent a radical nephrectomy. This patient's tissue was harvested, IFN treated, and three major signature IFN stimulated genes (ISGs), PKR, ISG 15K and ISG 56K, were investigated using real-time quantitative PCR.

Results and Conclusion: The index patient's normal and tumor kidney tissue was stimulated by IFN to increase transcription of all three genes. However, 6 of 7 other test patient's tumors revealed defects in at least one of the ISGs. This would translate into a 15% predicted response rate which agrees with clinical data. Molecular profiling of tissue may be prognostic in IFN responsiveness. A more accurate profile can be generated by using IFN stimulated gene chips that contain a larger number of ISGs and testing a larger number of patients who undergo nephrectomy prior to immunotherapy. This may allow not only the targeted treatment of IFN responsive patients but also avoid needless exposure to the majority who will not have a response. Ultimately, the genetic profiles of IFN responsive and unresponsive patients will generate mechanistic models of how IFN works in RCC and how we may convert resistance into IFN-responsiveness.

O-37

RELATIONSHIP BETWEEN PRETREATMENT HEMOGLOBIN LEVELS AND DISEASE RESPONSE, NEOANGIOGENESIS AND KI67 EXPRESSION IN BREAST CANCER PATIENTS UNDERGOING PRIMARY CHEMOTHERAPY

Daniele Generali, MD, Alberto Bottini, MD, Alfredo Berruti, MD, Alessandra Bersiga, MD, Maria Pia Brizzi, MD, Giovanni Allevi, MD, Sergio Aguggini, MD, Giovanna Bolsi, MD, Simone Bonardi, MD, Luigi Dogliotti, MD
Breast Unit, Azienda Ospedaliera Istituti Ospitalieri; Cremona, Oncologia Medica, Azienda Ospedaliera San Luigi, Orbassano, Italy

We investigated the impact of hemoglobin (Hb) levels on clinical and biological features in breast cancer patients receiving primary chemotherapy. From 1990 to 1997, 2 consecutive phase II studies of primary chemotherapy were conducted in our Institution. These studies involved 157 breast cancer patients with operable or locally advanced disease (T2-4N0-1M0). The first 76 received the CMF regimen + tamoxifen, the remaining 81 were submitted to single agent epirubicin. Tumor specimens were obtained before chemotherapy by incision biopsy and at definitive surgery, respectively. Tumor shrinkage (>50%) was obtained in 113 out of 156 evaluable cases (72.4%). Pathological complete response was attained in 3 (2%) cases. The mean Hb levels (+SD) at baseline conditions was 13.5 g/dl (+1.2) in responding patients and 13.13 (+1.0) in non-responders (p=0.06). The corresponding figures of red blood cell count (RBC) were 4.56 (+0.39) and 4.35 (+0.36), respectively (p <0.01). A cut off of 13 g/dl was defined to discriminate between normal and low Hb levels. Patients with a starting condition of low Hb levels obtained a lower response rate than their counterpart [36/61 (59.0%) vs 77/95 (81.0%), p < 0.003]. All patients attaining complete pathological response had normal pretreatment Hb. Ki 67 immunostaining at baseline condition did not differ comparing patients with low [median 14.5 (range 1-50)] or normal Hb [16.0 (range 1-90)], but low baseline Hb status was predicitve of higher Ki67 expression in post operative BC specimens [median 9.5 (range 0-80) vs 5 (range 0-50), p<0.03]. Blood microvessel count (MVC) by CD34 immunostaining were available before and after treatment in 120 matched pair breast cancer samples. There was a low but significant inverse relationship between Hb levels and MVC either before (Spearman r - 0.23) and after treatment (Spearman r - 0.24) (p<0.05). To conclude, baseline Hb status significantly predicted treatment response in breast cancer patients undergoing primary chemotherapy. Our data also suggest a possible contribution of Hb levels in influencing tumor-induced neoangiogenesis and antiproliferative effect of the cytotoxic treatment.

O-38

PAI-1 PROMOTER-DRIVEN PAI-1-GFP EXPRESSION VECTORS: TOOLS FOR ASSESSMENT OF TRANSCRIPTIONAL ACTIVITY AND CELLULAR INVASIVE TRAITS

Paul J. Higgins, PhD
Center for Cell Biology & Cancer Research, Albany Medical College, Albany, NY

Plasminogen activator inhibitor type-1 (PAI-1), the major regulator of plasmin generation, is required for tumor invasion and the angiogenic response. Plasmin is utilized by both tumor cells and activated endothelial cells to locomote through complex extracellular matrix/stromal tissue barriers. PAI-1 synthesis must be tightly controlled in these processes as deficient PAI-1 expression (as in the PAI-1-/- mouse) or excessive PAI-1 production is incompatible with maintenance of a matrix "scaffold" structure permissive for tumor invasion or formation of functional neocapillaries. To assess PAI-1 function in cell migration, 800 bp of the human PAI-1 promoter were cloned upstream of a GFP insert. PAI-1 transcription in transfectants was confirmed by Northern blotting and, at the single cell level, by GFP reporter activity after the switch from a sessile to motile phenotype. GFP expression was activated (as was the endogenous gene) within the real time of induced motility and only in the migrating cohort. To evaluate this relationship more directly, a second vector was developed in which 800 bp of the PAI-1 promoter was cloned upstream of an insert encoding a PAI-1-GFP chimeric protein. De novo-synthesized PAI-1-GFP was tracked in situ by fluorescence microscopy. Such PAI-1 expressing cells were highly motile in 2-D and 3-D migration assays. Moreover, invasive traits could be "rescued" in PAI-1-/- cells upon transfection with PAI-1/PAI-1-GFP expression vectors. The level of chimeric protein expressed correlated with cellular migratory activity and attenuation of PAI-1 synthesis by constitutive or inducible PAI-1 antisense vectors ablated the migratory response. These findings illustrate the usefulness of this approach to image transcriptional and migratory events in single cells using promoters from genes implicated in cellular invasive traits. Supported by grants from the NIH (GM57242) and the Department of the Army.

O-39

EFFICACY OF AN ANTI-SONIC HEDGEHOG MONOCLONAL ANTIBODY IN CANCER XENOGRAFT MODELS

Juliet A. Williams, PhD, Arlyssa LaPorte, Tim Racie, Yin Xu, Frank Y. Wang, PhD, David Bumcrot, PhD
Curis, Inc., Cambridge, MA

Tumor pathogenesis critically depends upon the interaction between cancer cells and the surrounding environment. Mutant cancer cell types can subvert normal cell types to produce factors necessary for processes such as angiogenesis, immune suppression and invasiveness. Several secreted signaling molecules responsible, at least in part for these activities have been identified, and moreover, therapeutic strategies aimed at inhibiting these signaling pathways have shown promise in the clinic.

Our studies have focused on the role of the Hh pathway in cancer. It has been established that activation of the Hh pathway by mutation is the causative event in Basal Cell Carcinoma and may play a role in other cancers. In addition, the discovery that Shh can induce angiogenic factors in fibroblasts indicates that Shh could also play a role in promoting cancer in the absence of activating pathway mutations.

Here we show many human cancer cell lines do indeed express Shh mRNA and produce active protein. Using several human cancer cell lines in xenograft mouse models, we demonstrate that Shh production is maintained in tumors in vivo and activates the hedgehog pathway in surrounding cells. We further show that systemic delivery of a monoclonal antibody directed against Shh causes a reduction in growth and in some cases regression of established tumors. These results significantly add to the importance of the Hh pathway and moreover the Shh ligand as a therapeutic target in cancer drug development.

O-40

PROGNOSTIC VALUE OF PREOPERATIVE SERUM CEA, CA19-9, CA242, CA72-4 AND HCGBETA IN PANCREATIC CANCER

Johanna Louhimo, MD, Anne Juuti, MD, Henrik Alfthan, PhD, Ulf-Håkan Stenman, MD, PhD,
Caj Haglund, MD, PhD
Department of Surgery and Department of Clinical Chemistry, University of Helsinki, Helsinki, Finland

Pancreatic cancer is one of the major causes of cancer related death in the western world with a low 5-year relative survival of only 4%. The aim of the study was to evaluate the prognostic significance of a panel of tumor markers (CEA, CA19-9, CA242, CA72-4 and hCGbeta) with preoperative serum samples from 125 patients (53 males and 72 females) with pancreatic cancer. Patients included 5 patients with stage I, 15 with stage II, 18 with stage III and 87 with stage IV histologically or cytologically proven pancreatic adenocarcinoma. The serum levels of CEA, CA19-9, CA242, and CA72-4 were measured with commercial kits (Wallac, Bayer, CanAg) with cut-off values of 5 ug/L for CEA, 37 kU/L for CA19-9, 20 kU/L for CA242, 6 kU/L for CA72-4. The serum hCGbeta was quantitated by an immunofluorometric assay (IFMA) based on our own monoclonal antibody with 2 pmol/L as a cut-off value.

The sensitivities of the studied tumor markers were 47% for CEA, 84% for CA19-9, 66% for CA242, 40% for CA72-4, and 66% for hCGbeta. No correlation was found between marker positivity and stage, except for CA72-4, with highest frequencies of elevated marker levels in advanced disease ($p = 0.008$). The overall 2-year survival was 8%, and in stage I, II, III, and IV cancers the 2-year survival was 20%, 8%, 13%, and 1%, respectively. Assessed with univariate Kaplan-Meier life-table analysis and log rank test, CA72-4 ($p = 0.020$) and hCGbeta ($p < 0.001$) had prognostic significance in pancreatic cancer; elevated serum values correlated with worse survival. With Cox multivariate regression analysis, the strongest prognostic factor was preoperative hCGbeta ($p < 0.001$), but also stage ($p = 0.043$) and CA72-4 ($p = 0.042$) provided independent prognostic information.

In conclusion, in pancreatic cancer, elevated preoperative serum levels of CA72-4 and hCGbeta correlate with poor outcome, and in multivariate analysis, hCGbeta was the strongest prognostic factor, but independent prognostic significance was observed also with stage and CA72-4.

O-41

HOW COULD DECISION SUPPORT SYSTEM BASED ON NON-LINEAR MODEL HELP TO INTERPRET TUMOR MARKER MEASUREMENTS IN ONCOLOGY

L. Pecen, K. Eben, J. Vondracek, L. Holubec , O. Topolcan, R. Pikner, J. Kausitz, M. Nekulova, M. Simickova
Institute of Computer Science, Prague, Czech Republic, Faculty Hospital Pilsen, Czech Republic, MOU Brno, Czech Republic, St. Elizabeth's Institute of Oncology, Slovakia

Examinations of tumor markers belong today to standard diagnostic methods. Most of these markers show pathological values in more diagnoses, several parameters being measured simultaneously. In the course of the patient´s illness, tumor markers are measured repeatedly, and it is useful to observe the dynamics of their development in time. Such and other circumstances have led to the beginning of co-operation between physicians and mathematicians, resulting in several mathematical models having been implemented into the respective programmes. The purpose of such models is effectively to make use of information contained in tumor markers together with some of clinical data and to summarise it as probabilities of particular illnesses and clinical status. Model parameters are estimated on the basis of statistical processing of a suitable reference file of patients, taking into consideration information from the literature and from experts in the given field. The models also take into account epidemiological data, in particular incidence and prevalence of illness. Correlations between laboratory parameters and their mutual influencing are also taken into consideration. The model output - quantified assessment of current and previous laboratory findings for the given patient - then becomes besides the clinical picture one of the components serving for the physician´s decision taking.

The question dealt with in the programme BIANTA is the determination of an unknown type and the location of primary tumor. The main task of the programme CRACTES is early diagnostics of the recurrence of tumor illness and its most probable location.

O-42

THE PREDICTIVE VALUE OF TRACE ELEMENTS IN SCREENING BREAST CANCER PATIENTS AT RISK OF DEVELOPING OVARIAN CANCER

Sawsan M.Rohaiem, Asmaa F. A. Sayed, Hesham A. M. Gomma
Physiology and Gynecology & Obstetric, Departments Faculty of Medicine and Biochemistry Department, Faculty of Pharmacy, Al Azhar University, Cairo, Egypt

It is commonly thought that the ovary is a preferable site for breast cancer metastasis. It is well established that nutritional excess or deficiencies could modify the susceptibility of the host tissue to a carcinogen. This study aims at testing the predictive value of an immunochemical panel to detect the breast cancer patients at risk of developing ovarian cancer. The efficacy of CA125, Cu, Zn, and Cu / Zn ratio are estimated. This study includes 190 patients, where they are divided into three groups; groups A (100 breast cancer non-smoking postmenopausal women), group B (50 non-smoking postmenopausal women with benign breast disease) and group C (40 healthy non-smoking postmenopausal women as control group). All patients have age range between (45-65 yrs with mean age 55.4 ±11.82 yrs). All patients are submitted to full history taking, clinical and pelvic examination and transvaginal ultrasonography. The operative biopsy from breast cancer and benign breast disease groups are submitted to histopathological examination. Follow up is carried out in the group of malignancy post-operatively and during the subsequent therapy with tamoxifen. CA125 is estimated by microparticle enzyme immunoassay (ABBOT Diagnostic. USA). Cu & Zn are analyzed by atomic absorption spectro-photometer. Eleven out of 100 breast cancer patients developed ovarian masses. Three of them proved to be malignant (3/100 = 3% & 3 /11 = 27 %), the remaining 8 cases are benign ovarian cysts (1-5 cm). The mean values of CA125 in normal, benign ovarian cysts, and ovarian cancer patients are respectively; 12.99 ±10.67, 57.74 ± 91.10 and 1058.75 ± 1843.92 u/ml ($p < 0.001$). The mean values for serum Cu in the three studied groups are respectively 0.96 ± 0.25, 1.27 ± 0.48 and 2.04 ± 0.49 mg/L ($p < 0.001$). The cut-off value of Cu is 2.05 mg/L to discriminate between the non-malignant and ovarian cancer groups. The values for serum Zn in the three mentioned groups are respectively 1.20 ± 0.58, 1.38 ± 0.43 and 0.47 ± 0.36 mg/L ($p < 0.001$). The cut-off value of Zn in this study is 0.34 mg/L. Cu/Zn ratio in the study groups are 1.005 ± 0.65, 1.06 ± 0.62 and 44.53 ± 72.48 respectively, with ($p < 0.01$), and the cut-off value is 2.30 %. Our study found that there is a correlation between Cu/Zn ratio and ovarian malignancy. Cu/Zn ratio served as a better biomarker especially when combined with CA125 as they give a high sensitivity of 96.1 % instead of 85 % for Cu/Zn ratio alone for the early detection of breast cancer patients susceptible to develop ovarian malignancy.

O-43

EVALUATION OF THE NEW CYFRA 21-1 URINE ASSAY FOR BLADDER CANCER

B. Nisman, D. Pode, D. Golijanin, A. Shapiro, T. Peretz, V. Barak
Oncology Department and Urology Department, Hadassah University Hosp, Jerusalem, Israel

Background: Cytokeratin 19 belongs to the intermediate filaments found in all epithelial cells. Its overexpression has been observed in malignant urothelial tumors. After cell lysis, it is released into urine in the form of soluble fragments measured by the CYFRA 21-1 assay.

Aims: To evaluate the non-invasive urine CYFRA 21-1 assay for early detection of primary and recurrent bladder cancer as well as to compare its efficacy to the standard urine cytology.

Patients and Methods: A prospective study was performed on urine samples from 342 subjects. 152 patients (pts) presented with hematuria or irritative voiding symptoms (group 1); 107 pts under surveillance, after transurethral resection of bladder cancer (group 2); 63 pts with urinary stones and infection (group 3) and 20 healthy subjects (group 4).

Results: The CYFRA 21-1 assay showed a sensitivity of 79.3% and a specificity of 88.6% for the detection of primary bladder tumors. For recurrent bladder tumors the assay sensitivity and specificity were 76.2% and 84.2%, respectively. The assay provided a 3-fold higher sensitivity than cytology for detection of grade 1 tumors. It identified 71% of primary and 65% of recurrent tumors, which were missed by urine cytology. Centrifugation of the urine samples or determination of the creatinine concentration in the urine samples did not improve the accuracy of the assay. Urinary stones, infection and previous intravesical BCG immunotherapy caused many false positive results (80%, 90.3% and 44% respectively).

Conclusions: The urinary CYFRA 21-1 is a useful assay for non-invasive detection of bladder cancer and for surveillance of pts not treated previously with BCG. It may be used in combination with cytology.

O-44

PROGNOSIS AND RESPONSE TO HERCEPTIN BY TUMOR MARKERS IN BREAST CANCER

V. Barak, B. Nisman, A. Hubert, O. Lyass, T. Peretz
Department of Oncology, Hadassah University Hospital, Jerusalem, Israel

Background: The circulating tumor mass markers CA15-3, CA125, CEA in breast cancer are well established. We have previoulsy shown that TPS (Cytokeratin 18) is a very sensitive marker of disease activity in breast cancer. The Her-2/neu serum marker as well as its therapy-Herceptin, are both available now for about 33% of breast cancers in which they are overexpressed.
Aims and Methods: To evaluate the prognostic potential of Tumor Markers (CA15-3, CA125, CEA, TPS) in 140 breast cancer Stage IV patients (pts) treated by Taxol following chemotherapy, monitored for 5 years. In addition, to compare TPS and Her-2/neu for the monitoring of Herceptin treated pts.
Results: A significant correlation of the marker levels with response, prognosis of remissions/recurrences (lead time - months) and survival, was demonstrated. Univariate analysis of pretreatment baseline marker levels showed significance for CA125, TPS and CEA only, but not for CA15-3. Median survival time of pts with pre-Taxol low levels of CA 125, TPS and CEA were 21.3 m, 16.7 m, 16,5 m as opposed to high marker levels; 9.1 m, 9.0 m, 9.7 m - respectively. Survival was best correlated to low CA 125 and TPS entering levels. CA125 and TPS retained significance also in the multivariate Cox's regression analysis, with relative risks of 2.3 and 2.1 vs 1. When higher cut off levels were defined by the recursive partitioning binary trees technique, all 4 markers were found as significant factors. CA125 and TPS were again independent prognosticators in the multivariate Cox's regression analysis, with relative risks of 2.7 and 1.7 vs 1. Response to Herceptin was monitored by serial determinations of Her-2/neu and TPS with a lead time of 4 -7 m indicating recurrence.
Conclusions: CA 125 and TPS provide the most important information for prognosis in advanced breast cancer pts treated by Taxol. Response to Herceptin treatment is efficiently monitored by both Her-2/neu and TPS, which provide prognostic information.

O-45

EVALUATION OF CEA, AFP AND CA 15-3: DIAGNOSTIC SIGNIFICANCE IN PATIENTS WITH GIT, HEPATOCELLULAR AND BREAST CARCINOMA

Junaid Mahmood Alam, Ishrat Sultana
Department of Biochemistry and Chemical Pathology, Liaquat National Postgraduate Medical Centre
Karachi, Pakistan

CEA molecule is an Oncodevelopment human tumor marker and a glycoprotein of MW 180 kDa, consisting of a single polypeptide chain. It is present in large quantities in adenocarcinoma of GIT and lung and thyroid and medullary carcinoma. AFP is also a glycoprotein of the fetus, major source being the liver and visceral abdomen of the yolk sac. It has a MW weight of 66 kDa and consists of a single polypeptide chain of 590 amino acids. It is one of the major oncofetal antigen present mainly in hepatocellular carcinoma. Moreover, another tumor marker, CA 15-3 is a mucin-like antigen, circulating in breast cancer patients. It is a glycoprotein of MW 300 kDa with two monoclonal antibodies, 115 D8 against milk fat membrane and DF 3 against breast carcinoma cell line. Presently, the major clinical applications include the pre-clinical detection of breast carcinoma recurrence, assessment of its prognosis and monitoring of therapy during treatments. In present study, serum CEA, AFP and CA 15-3 levels were determined in patients diagnosed with or suspected of malignancies and non-malignant conditions. A total of 403 test (patients) and 50 control (healthy) samples were analyzed on Cobas-Core (Roche Diagnostics, Basil) using ELISA techniques with full-calibrations and two point controls possessing defined cut-off values. Out of these 403, 150 (*46.60% males, 53.30% females*) were screened for CEA, of which 40% females gave marked elevated values whereas only 8-12% males share similar elevated pattern. Elevated CEA concentration in females corresponds to breast carcinoma, ovarian tumors and a few related non-malignant conditions and in males, mostly gastric and GIT carcinoma. Out of 178 patients (*60.60% males; 39.32% females*) examined for AFP, more than 50% exhibited elevated levels, which corresponds to their malignant (70-80%, hepatocellular and testicular carcinoma, germ cell tumor) and non-malignant (20%-30%, liver cirrhosis, hepatitis) conditions. Similarly, 59 (78.66%) out of 75 patients (all females) screened for CA 15-3, exhibited elevated levels and corresponds with breast carcinoma at various degree of malignancy. Only 16 (21.33%) were devoid of any malignant condition and diagnosed with ovarian cysts, breast lesions, GIT aberration and liver cirrhosis. The primary aim of the study was to correlate the abnormal levels of these circulating makers with a number of clinical and biological parameters, such as disease extent, age and types of metastases.

O-46

MICROARRAY MOLEOULAR PROFILING OF RENAL CELL CARCINOMA; MOLECULAR PATTERNS IN RCC AND THE ELUCIDATION OF PROGNOSTIC MARKERS IN PATIENTS

Louis S. Liou, MD, Provash Sadhukan, PhD, Elias Castilla, MD, Marek Skacel, MD,
Joseph DiDonato, PhD, Richard Babayan, MD, Andrew Novick, MD
Cleveland Clinic Foundation, Cleveland Heights, OH; Boston University Medical Center, Boston, MA

Renal cell carcinoma is the third most prevalent genito-urinary cancer. Surgical treatment is the standard of care and allows the pathological diagnosis of the disease. Some characteristics of the primary tumor have been described to correlate with poor clinical outcome and although the literature has many molecular marker proteins, there is not a molecular marker(s) that can portend a patient's clinical outcome. We utilized expression microarray technology to elucidate potential molecular markers of RCC clear cell type and determine correlation with clinical outcome in a tissue microarray. We found that comparing the expression profiles of 6 patient tumors (varying grades of clear cell RCC) and their matched normal tissue, a total of 80 genes were found to be up-regulated in the tumor. One highly expressed gene's protein product, neuron specific enolase, was found by immunohistochemistry to be expressed in 66% of a RCC tissue microarray but there was no correlation with tumor grade, stage, size, and patient outcome. Cyclo-oxygenase 2 gene message was not increased in the tumor but antibody staining did show an overall 26% positivity with a correlation to tumor stage and grade. Utilizing this approach, the disease of RCC can be dissected to the basic molecular level and will give us an in depth understanding of the pathobiology.

O-47

A GENOMIC SCREEN FOR GENES UPREGULATED BY DEMETHYLATION AND HDAC INHIBITION IN HUMAN COLORECTAL CANCER

Hiromu Suzuki, MD, PhD, Edward Gabrielson, MD, Wei Chen, James G. Herman, MD, Kohzoh Imai, MD, PhD, Stephen B. Baylin, MD; Sidney Comprehensive Cancer Center, Johns Hopkins University, Baltimore, MD; Sapporo Medical University, Sapporo, Japan

Aberrant hypermethylation of gene promoters is now recognized as one of the major mechanisms to inactivate tumor suppressor genes in cancer. We have previously shown that the transcriptional silencing associated with this DNA change is mediated by both the promoter methylation and histone de-acetylase activity (HDAC), with the methylation being dominant. Thus, the HDAC inhibitor, trichostatin (TSA) will not alone allow reexpression of hypermethylated tumor suppressor genes but will enhance such reexpression following minimal demethylation produced by low dose 5-aza-2′ deoxycytidine (DAC). In the present study, we have used a combination of cDNA subtraction followed by microarray analysis to screen for genes upregulated by low dose DAC and TSA treatment in a human colorectal cancer (CRC) cell line. From a total of 10,814 genes examined by subtraction microarray, we found 74 upregulated genes by DAC and/or TSA treatment. According to the subsequent analysis by semi-quantitative RT-PCR, we could divide those genes into two groups. Group 1 (n = 51) genes showed no change in expression with TSA alone, minimal increase in expression following low dose DAC alone, but much stronger induction by the combined DAC and TSA. Group 1 genes could be subdivided into two groups; group 1a genes (n = 24) are completely inactivated in mock cells, while group 1b genes (n = 27) show some basal expression detected by RT-PCR. Group 2 genes (n = 23), in contrast, are characterized by showing upregulation by TSA alone, and having a variable initial expression or response to DAC alone. We next performed methylation analysis of those genes that have already identified 5′ CpG islands. We found complete hypermethylation in 10 of 10 group 1a genes, and partial hypermethylation in 3 of 5 group 1b genes. However, none of the group 2 genes investigated showed any methylation, even though they have dense CpG islands around their transcription start sites. This screening strategy appears to be the most robust for identifying methylation changes specific to gene promoters and for identifying new tumor-related genes. We found hypermethylation in numerous genes with high potential for important roles in human cancers, including those encoding blockers of the WNT oncogene pathway, membrane receptors, regulators of calcium ion distribution, folate metabolism, cell adhesion, and RNA splicing.

O-49

PROGNOSTIC AND DIAGNOSTIC UTILITY OF GENE PROFILING OF BLADDER TUMORS

Marta Sanchez-Carbayo, PhD, Nicholas Socci, PhD, Juan Lozano, PhD, Wentian Li, PhD, Thomas Belbin, PhD, Michael Prystowski, MD, PhD, Angel Ortiz, PhD, Geoffrey Childs, PhD, Carlos Cordon-Cardo, MD, PhD
Memorial Sloan Kettering Cancer Center, Rockefeller University, Mount Sinai School of Medicine, Albert Einstein College of Medicine, New York, NY

The transcriptome of bladder tumors was compared against a pool of bladder cancer cell lines using cDNA microarrays. Hierarchical clustering combined with non-parametric bootstrap resampling techniques identified two clusters segregated superficial from invasive transitional carcinomas and provided prognostic information. Genes differentially expressed between superficial and invasive tumors were identified by Wilcoxon test, single logistic regression, and multidimensional techniques. Cytokeratin 20, neuropilin 2, p21, cyclin E, ninjurin and p33ING1 were selected among the top ranked molecular targets and validated by immunohistochemistry using tissue microarrays containing bladder tumors. The expression of these molecular targets was associated with histopathological stage, tumor grade and related to altered p53 and RB expression. Moreover, p33ING1 was associated with overall survival. A generated support vector machine revealed that WNT5a and mitotic spindle checkpoint are among the altered pathways during bladder cancer progression. Gene profiling classified bladder tumors based on their histopathogenesis and clinical outcome. Identified molecular targets were associated with tumor progression and survival in primary bladder tumors and might become useful markers to further stratify bladder cancer.

O-50

SYNAPTOPODIN AND MYOPODIN AS PROGRESSION MARKERS IN BLADDER CANCER

Marta Sanchez-Carbayo, PhD, Karin Schwartz, PhD, Christian Faul, Laura Barisoni, PhD, Gero von Gersdorff, MD, Elizabeth Charytonowicz, Geoffrey Childs, PhD, Peter Mundel, MD, PhD, Carlos Cordon-Cardo, MD, PhD
Memorial Sloan Kettering Cancer Center, Albert Einstein College of Medicine, New York, NY

We identified a differential expression of synaptopodin in bladder cancer in two gene profiling studies using cDNA microarrays. The expression profiling of nine bladder cancer cell lines versus a pool containing equal total RNA quantities of each of them revealed a loss in the expression of synaptopodin in the cells obtained from the most advanced bladder tumors as compared to the ones obtained from papillary tumors. When comparing 15 bladder tumors versus a pool of four bladder cancer cell lines, transcripts of synaptopodin were more abundant in normal urothelia and superficial than in invasive and metastatic tumors. In order to validate the clinical impact of this these genes in bladder cancer we analyzed the protein expression patterns of synaptopodin and its homologue myopodin in tissue microarrays of bladder tumors (n=173) by immunohistochemistry. The expression of synaptopodin and myopodin in the nuclei was found to be significantly associated with histopathological stage and grade in this subset of patients ($p<0.001$). In primary tumors, expression of these genes was also significantly related to altered RB expression and other markers related to p53-RB pathways. We also evaluated the association of myopodin with cell cycle by flow cytometry and sorting analysis as well as its prognostic value. Overall, gene expression profiling identified the potential involvement of novel molecular targets in bladder cancer. The expression patterns of synaptopodin and myopodin were shown to be involved in bladder cancer progression and might become useful markers to further stratify bladder tumors.

O-51

BREAST CANCER SUBTYPES IDENTIFIED BY USING cDNA MICROARRAYS ARE ROBUST ACROSS TWO INDEPENDENT DATASETS

Therese Sørlie, PhD, Robert Tibshirani, PhD, Anne-Lise Børresen-Dale, PhD, David Botstein, PhD
Department of Genetics, Department of Health Research and Policy, and Statistics, Stanford University, Stanford, CA; Department of Genetics, The Norwegian Radium Hospital, Oslo, Norway

We have classified 110 breast cancer cases, the majority of them stage III/IV with and without lymph node infiltration into five subgroups: basal epithelial, ERBB2+, normal breast-like and two luminal epithelial groups. The classification was based on variation in expression patterns of 550"intrinsic" genes, which were selected by their similar gene expression levels within samples obtained from the same tumor and variation across the different tumors. The subtypes showed significant differences in overall survival and time to relapse in Kaplan-Meier analyses. In order to investigate the robustness and validity of these tumor subgroups, we extracted data from an independent study on expression profiling of breast cancer (van't Veer et. al., Nature 415, 530-536, 2002). The same five groups of tumors appeared when gene expression values were extracted for 350 of the intrinsic genes and analyzed by hierarchical clustering. Moreover, when clustering our breast cancer samples using expression data for 67 of the 231 prognostic marker genes identified by van't Veer et al., we were able to recapitulate their two prognostic signature groups. The poor prognosis patients largely coincided with patients in the basal, ERBB2+ and Luminal B subgroups, whereas the patients with the good prognosis signature were predominantly the same as those in the Luminal A group. Our results suggest that these five subtypes are robust and inherent to breast cancer despite clinical and histopathological differences between the tumors. They also support the concept that multidimensional variation in gene expression patterns identified by cDNA microarrays can provide a platform for an improved classification scheme in breast cancer.

0-52

INTRATUMORAL EFFECTS OF LOW DOSE RADIATION AT RADIOIMMUNOTHERAPY

Torgny Stigbrand, David Eriksson, Homa I. Mirzaie J, Ali Sheikholvaezin, Per-Olov Löfroth, Katrine Riklund Åhlström, Lennart Johansson
Department of Immunology, Umeå University, Department of Radiation Sciences, Sections of Oncology, Radiation physics and Diagnostic Radiology, Umeå, Sweden

The intratumoral effects of low dose (2 – 5 Gy), low dose rate (0.045 Gy/h) g-irradiation as observed at experimental radioimmunotherapy are complex processes affecting cell proliferation, vascularization, tissue morphology and induction of apoptosis. Human HeLa Hep 2 carcinoma cells have been investigated in vitro and in vivo immunohistochemically with stainings for Ki67, M30, CD105, (endoglin) TUNEL, Annexin. Also DNA laddering and clonogenicity were investigated. The cells were exposed to low doses of g-radiation (i.e. 0.5, 1, 2, 5, 10, 15 Gy), by ^{60}Co using GAMMATRON3 and ALCYON2. Such radiation doses can be achieved by radioimmunotherapy. DNA strand-nicks were detected by the TUNEL staining and changes on the cell surface by ANNEXIN-V-FLUOS. FACS analysis and fluorescence microscopy were used to quantify apoptosis. Radiation doses below 2 Gy did not cause any significant apoptosis, but in the interval 5 – 15 Gy significant apoptosis was observed, with peak values at 5 Gy. Up to 60% of investigated cells were shown to display apoptosis. Time to this peak value was 168 hours after radiation The in vivo experiments revealed significant changes in tissue morphology, connective tissue distribution and apperance of of microvacuolization. It is concluded that low dose radiation can cause significant complex abberations in tumor cell growth including significant apoptosis apoptosis.

O-53

GENERATION AND IMMUNOCHEMICAL CHARACTERIZATION OF HUMAN MONOCLONAL ANTIBODIES TO CARCINOEMBRYONIC ANTIGEN (CEA)

Masahide Kuroki, MD, PhD, Takayuki Imakiire, MD, Motomu Kuroki, PhD, Hirotomo Shibaguchi, PhD
Department. of Biochem., Fukuoka University School of Medicine, Fukuoka, Japan

To reduce the immunogenicity of mouse monoclonal antibodies (mMAbs) in humans, genetically recombinant antibodies such as mouse/human chimeric antibody, humanized antibody or scFv antibody have been prepared to date. However, these antibodies are still weakly immunogenic in humans. In this study, we generated fully human monoclonal antibodies (hMAbs) to CEA by using the KM mouse (the Crossbred TransChromo mouse) and the usual hybridoma technique.

46 hybridoma clones producing hMAbs to CEA were prepared by fusions of the P3-U1 mouse myeloma cells with splenocytes of the KM mice immunized with purified CEA. Their specificities were systematically analysed by flow cytometry for reactivity with four CEA gene family members; CEA, NCA (CEACAM6), BGP (CEACAM1), and CGM6 (CEACAM8). Among them, the Group I hMAbs (22 clones) reacted only with CEA. 7 of the Group I hMAbs were of the IgG4(k), 2 were of the IgG3(k), one was IgG2(k), another was of the IgG1(k), and the remaining clones were not determined. The affinity constants for CEA of the Group I hMAbs were comparable to those of mMAbs previously prepared by ourselves. BIAcore analysis furthermore revealed that the Group I hMAbs were subdivided into 8 subgroups. When compared to 9 mMAbs with well defined specificity, 5 of the Group I hMAbs significantly competed with one of 4 mMAbs, respectively, implying that 4 of the Group I hMAbs recognized the epitopes on the domain N of the CEA molecule and one is reactive with that on the domain I. In in vitro experiments using human LAK cells, 4 Group I hMAbs tested exhibited 40 to 65% ADCC against CEA-expressing tumor cells. These results demonstrate that the nonimmunogenic Group I hMAbs may be useful for tumor imaging by immunoscintigraphy as well as for immunotherapeutic approaches.

O-54

PHOTODYNAMIC DIAGNOSIS OF PRIMARY TUMORS AND METASTASES IN MOUSE MAMMARY CARCINOMA

Heinrich Walt, PhD, Ann M. Dorward, PhD, Wesley G. Beamer, PhD
University Hospital, Zurich, Switzerland

Transgenic mouse models of mammary cancer have proven themselves as useful tools for investigating genetic contributions to neoplasia, as well as acting as models of human disease for testing various therapeutic modalities. In clinical practice it has been shown that primary human breast cancer can be discerned from surrounding normal tissues following oral consumption of the heme precursor aminolevulinic acid (ALA) (Ladner, DP et al., BJC 84:33-37, 2001). ALA is rapidly metabolized by the tumor cells into the fluorescent molecule protoporphyrin IX (PPIX), which makes the tumor fluoresce red when illuminated by 400nm light. We have tested this method of photodynamic diagnosis (PDD) in multiple mouse models of breast cancer to investigate the generality of this finding in tumor specimens of different histological and genetic backgrounds, and to test the limits of PDD to demarcate tumor margins. Multiple mouse strains with spontaneous, palpable mammary tumors were examined for ALA to PPIX conversion following tail vein injection of the ALA precursor (100mg/kg, ASAT AG, Zug, Switzerland). These tumors arose in transgenic mouse strains with directed expression of oncogenic proteins in the mammary epithelium (HRAS, NEU, Polyoma virus T antigen (PyVT), and SV40 Large T antigen (WAPTag), or via infection with mammary tumor virus. In this strain survey, each tumor could be positively identified macroscopically by moderate to strong PPIX fluorescence intensity under 400nm light when examined in situ,1-2hrs post ALA injection. The finding that rapid PPIX conversion was a general property of mouse mammary tumors irrespective of oncogenic stimulus or genetic background (C3H/HeJ, FVB/N or C57BL/6J) was a similar conclusion to that reported in the preliminary human study. In addition, we were able to discern a lung metastasis originating from a mammary tumor of a PyVT female, and early hyperplastic lesions in mammary glands of a WAPTag female. Our preliminary experiments have confirmed that strategies for ALA-mediated PDD can be further investigated and optimized in mouse models of breast cancer, and these advances should be directly translatable to human clinical practice.

O-55

THYMALFASIN UP-REGULATES TUMOR ANTIGEN EXPRESSION IN COLORECTAL CANCER CELLS

Paola Sinibaldi-Vallebona, PhD, Pasquale Pierimarchi, MD, Gabriella Moroni, PhD, AnnaLucia Serafino, PhD, Maria Pia Fuggetta, PhD, Cynthia Tuthill, PhD, Guido Rasi, MD
University "Tor Vergata", Rome, CNR Institute of Neurobiology and Molecular Medicine, Rome, SciClone Pharmaceuticals, Inc., San Mateo, CA

Background: The development of anticancer vaccines, immuno-imaging and drug delivery techniques all depend on the identification of specific molecular targets (e.g., tumor antigens) that are available at the tumor cell membrane and are properly presented by MHC-1 molecules. Previously we have shown that TLP, a tumor specific antigen, is expressed in both human and experimental tumors, and has a conserved sequence. Thymalfasin, a 28 amino-acid immuno-stimulatory peptide, has been shown to up-regulate MHC-1 expression. In the present study we evaluated whether thymalfasin is able to up-regulate the expression of TLP on colorectal cancer cells, either in vitro or in vivo. **Methods:** (1) WiDr (human), IA-XsSBR (rat), and DHD-K12 (rat) colorectal cancer cell lines were treated with thymalfasin from 6 to 48 hours at 5 - 50 ug/ml. TLP antigen expression was determined by flow cytometry (FC) and antigen localization by confocal laser scanning microscopy (CLSM), using TLP antiserum raised against a 9 amino acid peptide epitope of TLP (CSH-237). (2) BD-IX rats were injected i.p. with syngeneic DHD-K12 cells and treated i.p. with thymalfasin. TLP expression and localization were determined as above on tumor cells obtained from ascites. **Results:** (1) TLP is naturally expressed in all 3 colorectal cell lines, both in the cytoplasm, ranging from 30-55% of cells (by CLSM and by FC after permeabilization) and on the cell membrane, ranging from 10-20% of cells (by FC). Thymalfasin is able to enhance the expression of this antigen in all cell lines. The level of enhancement, and localization at the membrane versus the cytoplasm, varies with dosage and timing of treatment, and can reach expression levels of 90% of cells. (2) Tumor cells in ascites from animals treated with thymalfasin demonstrate a similar enhancement of expression of TLP. **Conclusions:** The expression of TLP antigen can be up-regulated by treatment with thymalfasin. The increased expression could lead to more effective CTL responses from induction of a specific CD8 population. Additionally, this increased expression could allow cells to be better targeted and detected for radio-immuno guided surgery or immuno-scintigraphic techniques. Moreover, the availability of an experimental tumor naturally expressing a human antigen could be of great use in development of preclinical models. The ability to enhance the expression of a tumor antigen with a non-toxic treatment such as thymalfasin could thus be quite useful for both therapeutic and diagnostic purposes.

O-56

TUMOR INTRAVASATION IS VASCULOGENESIS TURNED INSIDE OUT

Sanford H. Barsky, MD and Mary L. Alpaugh, PhD
Department of Pathology, UCLA School of Medicine, Los Angeles, CA

The step of tumor intravasation is considered a rate-limiting step in spontaneous metastasis yet the molecular mechanisms of this step have not been clearly elucidated. We have developed a human inflammatory breast carcinoma / scid mouse xenograft model (MARY-X) which exhibits an exaggerated degree of intravasation characterized by florid lymphovascular emboli within both lymphatics as well as blood vessels. 30% of the xenograft consists of murine mesenchyme and vessels. The xenograft gives rise to spheroids in suspension culture which are 98-99% human but when reinjected into mice faithfully reproduce the MARY-X phenotype of florid lymphovascular tumor emboli. Green fluorescence protein (GFP)-labelled murine embryonal fibroblasts co-injected with purified spheroids reproduce the MARY-X phenotype and a strongly fluorescing xenograft in which the GFP is present within the tumoral stroma and the endothelial cells which surround the tumor emboli. Injected GFP-labelled spheroids also reproduce the MARY-X phenotype and a strongly fluorescing xenograft but one in which the GFP is present only within the tumor cells and not the tumoral stroma nor the surrounding endothelial cells. GFP-labelled adult stem cells derived from adipose tissue co-injected with purified spheroids reproduce the MARY-X phenotype but a non-fluorescing xenograft in which GFP is not detected in either tumor cells, stroma or endothelial cells. Two derived mutants of MARY-X, one containing a dominant negative E-cadherin mutant (H-2K^d-E-cad) which disrupts the E-cadherin-mediated homotypic adhesion of the spheroids and the other containing "-1,3-fucosyltransferase III (FucT-III), an enzyme which increases surface sialyl $Lewis^{x/a}$ which also disrupts the E-cadherin-mediated homotypic adhesion of the spheroids, both lose the MARY-X phenotype. When these mutant spheroids are co-injected with GFP-labelled murine embryonal fibroblasts, GFP is not detected in either tumor cells, stroma or surrounding endothelial cells. Our studies indicate that tumor intravasation may be a manifestation of vasculogenesis turned inside out because the tumor embolus stimulates the vascular channel to form around it. This occurs only if the right effector cell(s), ie. the intact tumoral spheroid and the right target cells with vasculogenesis potential are present. The direct origin of the so-called vasculogenic mimicry is not tumor cells but host mesenchymal (stem) cells.

O-57

NEWLY DEVELOPED CYTOKERATIN ANTIBODY AND ITS CORRELATION TO CLINICAL PARAMETERS IN NON-SMALL CELL LUNG CANCER PATIENTS

Michael Bergqvist, MD, Daniel Brattström, MD, Patrik Hesselius, Gunnar Wagenius, MD, Ola Brodin, MD
Department of Oncology, Radiology and Clinical Immunology, Uppsala University Hospital, Uppsala, Sweden

Background: Cytokeratins are of interest in human malignancies due to its function as building stones in the cytoskeleton of individual cells. In this study, we have investigated a newly developed monoclonal assay, MonoTotal TM, in which the monoclonal antibodies used are directed to various epitopes on cytokeratin 8, 18 and 19. **Objectives:** To investigate, in apparently healthy controls, the cut-off value for MonoTotal TM according to the 95 % lognormal distribution. To correlate data from the MonoTotal TM with clinical parameters in patients with non-small cell lung cancer. **Methods:** Patients with a histopathologically confirmed diagnosis of non-small cell lung cancer (NSCLC) were investigated for the presence of MonoTotal TM(a two-site monoclonalimmunoradiometric (sandwich) assay). These patients were followed from time of diagnosis until time of death and donated continuously serum samples that were stored at -70 C until analysed. A total of 300 apparently healthy Swedish blood donor individuals were investigated for the presence of MonoTotal TM. The study was approved by the research ethical committee at Uppsala University. **Results:** A total of 438 serum samples from seventy-two patients were included. In this study, the range of MonoTotal TM was 15.7-2252.0 U/l. The cut-off value was decided to 60 U/l according to the 95 % lognormal distribution in healthy blood donors. At time of diagnosis, 69 of the patients included in this study had elevated levels (>60 U/l) of MonoTotal TM. The higher the value was for MonoTotal TM at time of diagnosis, the poorer was the prognosis (p=0.0022). No statistical difference was found between median value of MonoTotal TM and staging according to TNM, histological subgroups, smoking habits, classification according to Zubrod. From time of diagnosis until death, a median increase 705 U/l of MonoTotal TM found and during radiation treatment, a statistical decrease in MonoTotal TM was found (p=0.0021). **Conclusion:** MonoTotal TM, in conjunction with other clinical data, give the clinician additive information concerning the prognosis of the individual patient at time of diagnosis.

O-58

A NEW IMMUNOASSAY FOR S100B PROTEIN

Ylva D'Amico, Lotta Hirschberg, PhD, Ingrid Davidsson
AB Sangtec Medical, Bromma, Sweden

The calcium binding protein S100B is expressed in melanocytes and in astroglia cells, as a dimmer. The family of S100 proteins contain 19 members. Patients with progressive melanoma disease show elevated serum concentrations of S100B. Continuing measurement of S100B is therefore a tool for monitoring melanoma patients. The protein is also shown to be a marker of brain damage and is released in blood. The clinical value of the chemiluminometric technique has been demonstrated in stroke, in cerebral complications in association with cardiac arrest and in patients with severe as well as minor head injury.

We have used this technique to develope a new ELISA assay for the detection of S100B (Sangtec100® ELISA) in serum and liquor samples. The ELISA is a one-step sandwich assay with an incubation time of 2 hours and a total assay time of less than 3 hours for a 48 sample microtitre plate. The required sample volume is 50 µl. For the detection we use HRP conjugated Ab and TMB substrate. The detection limit for the ELISA is 0,01 µg/L. The upper limit of the measuring range is 5 µg/L. The precision is below 10% within assay and below 5% between assays. The recovery when diluting samples is in average 96%. No high dose hook effect is detected in concentrations up to 5000 µg/L.

O-59

COMPARATIVE ANALYSIS OF LDH AND SERUM S-100B AS MARKERS OF DISEASE PROGRESSION IN THE FOLLOW UP OF MELANOMA PATIENTS

Axel Hauschild, MD, Wolfgang Hitschler, MD, Clemens Nitschke, MD, Stephan Lischner, MD, Enno Christophers, MD
Department of Dermatology, University of Kiel, Kiel, Germany

The new melanoma staging classification system (AJCC 2002) has incorporated a serum marker (LDH) for the first time as a relevant prognostic factor in stage IV advanced melanoma. We were interested to assess the value of LDH blood levels compared to serum concentrations of S-100B, a protein well known to be expressed in virtually all melanomas using immunohistology.

Therefore, a prospective study on 98 melanoma patients with intermediate- and high-risk of relapse (greater than 1.5mm tumor thickness and/or lymph node metastasis) was performed. During the observation period of 30 months 52 patients (53.1%) demonstrated disease progression. The clinical course of disease had been correlated to changes of LDH- and S-100B serum concentrations. The following results have been obtained: a) neither LDH or S-100B were indicators of in-transit metastases, b) the detection of clinically apparent lymph nodes succeeded in a minority of patients using LDH (11.8%) or S-100B (35.3%) only and c) the S-100B assessment (50.0%) was clearly superior to LDH (15.4%) in the identification of early distant metastases. The rate of false-positive (elevated) LDH and S-100B serum levels in currently disease-free melanoma patients did not differ significantly between the two markers (S-100B, 13.0% vs. LDH, 10.9%).

In conclusion, the study indicates that only S-100B serum concentration changes are relatively sensitive and specific markers for early melanoma macrometastases, but both markers are not able to identify occult micrometastases in high-risk melanoma patients. In the meantime a prospective study on the value of clinical examinations, technical evaluations and blood-testing in the routine follow-up of 4000 melanoma patients following standard surgery has been initiated. The measurement of S-100B serum concentrations has been referred into routine in many dermatologic centers.

O-60

COMPARISON OF LEVELS OF THE ONCOOVARIAN ANTIGENS CA-125 AND SOVA-1 IN SOME BIOLOGICAL FLUIDS OF HUMAN

Petr G. Prokopenko, MD, PhD, Svetlana A. Borisenko, MD, Albert V. Sokolov, MD, Alexander A. Terentiev, MD, PhD
Department of Biochemistry and Department of Obstetrics and Gynecology of the Russian State Medical University, Moscow, Russia

To date, the problem of early diagnostic of ovarian cancer is at the position that it was 30 years ago. Approximately 80% of women diagnosed with ovarian cancer are already at the high stage (III-IV) of the disease at their initial therapy. During last 30 years neither diagnosis nor 5-year survival have greatly improved for these patients. Thus "ovarian cancer remains the number one killer of women with gynecologic malignant hyperplasia" (Tanimoto H. et al., 2001). This is substantially due to absent of good tumor marker for early diagnosis of ovarian cancer. CA-125 is good tumor marker for monitoring but not for diagnosis of ovarian cancer. After the isolation of poor preparation CA-125 (Yin B.M. & Lloyd K.O., 2001) with activity 7 MU/mg it has become clear that CA-125 is normal tissue antigen - the glycoprotein (mucin-MUC16). As a rule the level of CA-125 in the healthy peoples serum is 35-65 MU/ml that correspondes to 5-9 mg/L. In classic immunochemistry suchlike antigens are regarded as normal minor serum components. The article studies comparison levels of the CA-125 and SOVA-1 in some biological fluids of the healthy people and ovarian cancer patients. SOVA-1 was prepared from serum of ovarian cancer patients. It is olygomer that consists of subunits (monomers) with Mm 36 kD. On SDS denatured electrophoresis the monomers are dissociating at polypeptide chains with Mm 18 kD. SOVA-1 has property to organize the olygomers: three-, tetra- and pentamers. The level of SOVA-1 in the serum of the healthy peoples is lower 50 mg/L (CA-125 - about 5-9 mg/L). SOVA-1 is not immunochemical identic with known oncofetal, placental and reactant proteins. In serum of ovarian cancer patients SOVA-1 is found in 75% cases (69% - I-II stage and 76% - III-IV stage of disease) with level of 1-10 mg/L, whereas level CA-125 may achieve 150-200 mg/L in serum and 1-1.5 g/L in ascytic fluid of ovarian cancer patients. SOVA-1 in contradistinction to CA-125 was not revealed in the ascytic fluid. In amniotic fluid its level is 50-100 mg/L. SOVA-1 is revealed in extracts from oncoovarian tissues, it is found in 25% cases of patients with non-malignant ovarian tumor and other cancer localization (uterus, stomach, small intestine).

O-61

IN-VITRO MATURATION OF HIGH AFFINITY SINGLE-CHAIN FV ANTIBODIES AGAINST TUMOUR ANTIGENS

Christian Fermér, PhD, Olle Nilsson, PhD, Karin Nilsson
CanAg DIagnostics AB, Gothenburg, Sweden

High affinity monoclonal antibodies (mAbs) with specificity for tumour antigens are by tradition successfully produced by conventional hybridoma technology. However, certain antigen molecules fail to produce an adequate immune response and thus only low affinity mAbs are produced. The possibility to clone the variable regions of antibodies and display them on the surface on phage as single-chain Fv antibody fragments (scFvs) opens the possibility to improve the affinity or in fact any characteristics, as long it's selectable, by in vitro maturation. In this study, high affinity scFvs against pro-gastrin-releasing peptide (pro-GRP), an antigen proven useful as a marker for small cell lung cancer, were derived from spleen cells of immunized mice and from hybridoma cell lines secreting low affinity antibodies. Repertoires of mutant variants were generated from the initial low affinity scFvs by an in-vitro recombination method, DNA shuffling, a technique that both introduces new mutations as well as links existing ones into new combinations. ScFv antibody fragments with improved affinity to pro-GRP, extracted from the libraries after several rounds of biopanning, were used as templates for construction of additional mutant libraries. The stepwise increase in affinity was carefully monitored by plasmon surface resonance (BIAcore) studies and nucleotide sequence analyses could link the improved affinities to specific mutations most often located in the complementarity determining regions (CDRs) in the heavy or light chain variable segments.

In vitro maturated single-chain Fv antibodies have the potential to be used directly in ELISA assays as diagnostic tools or might be further processed into functional human monoclonal antibodies and thus be a source of mAbs for use in human therapy.

O-62

INDUCTION OF MULTIPLE MYELOMA-SPECIFIC CYTOTOXIC T LYMPHOCYTES

Toshiaki Hayashi, MD, PhD, Teru Hideshima, MD, PhD, Nikhil C. Munshi, MD, Kohzoh Imai, MD, PhD, Kenneth C. Anderson, MD
The Jerome Lipper Multiple Myeloma Center, Dana-Farber Cancer Institute, Boston, MA, First Department of Internal Medicine, Sapporo Medical University School of Medicine, Sapporo, Japan

Background & Aims: Multiple myeloma (MM) remains an incurable plasma cell malignancy. However, recent studies show that allogeneic stem cell transplant may achieve prolonged progression-free survival compared to autografting, and that donor leukocyte infusion is effective in relapsed MM patients after bone marrow transplantation. These reports suggest that an immune-mediated allogeneic graft versus myeloma effect is inducible, providing the framework for promising immune-based therapeutic options. In this study, we investigate the strategy for inducing MM-specific cytotoxic T lymphocytes (CTL) by vaccination. **Methods:** Immature dendritic cells (DCs) were induced by culture of adherent mononuclear cells in the presence of GM-CSF and IL-4. After pulsing with apoptotic bodies generated by irradiation of MM cells, immature DCs were cultured with TNF-£ to induce maturation. PBMC from the same donor were then stimulated with the apoptotic MM body-pulsed DCs weekly. Seven days after the second stimulation, cytotoxicity of the CTL was examined against the tumor cell used for stimulation with DC, as well as against unrelated MM cells, to confirm specificity of response. To characterize the CTL, flow cytometric analysis and target blocking assays using anti-HLA class I and II antibodies were performed. **Results:** T cells stimulated by this method showed higher proliferation than those stimulated by tumor cells only, DCs only, or tumor lysate-pulsed DCs. The CTLs showed specific cytotoxicity to the MM cells used to pulse DC for stimulation. Phenotypic analysis revealed that these cells were CD3- and CD8-positive and CD56-negative. Moreover, target blocking assays using HLA class I or class II antibodies showed that cytotoxicity of the CTLs was HLA-class I-restricted. **Conclusion:** This strategy may allow generation of CTL from patients, regardless of the expression of a certain tumor antigens or HLA types, and therefore offer novel immunotherapy to improve patient outcome in MM.

O-63

INDUCTION OF TUMOR- AND CA125- SPECIFIC IFN-GAMMA ELISPOT RESPONSES IN OVARIAN CANCER PATIENTS TREATED WITH OREGOVOMAB CORRELATE WITH IMPROVED TIME TO RELAPSE AND SURVIVAL

Birgit C. Schultes, PhD, Alan Gordon, MD, Christopher F. Nicodemus, MD, Robert Edwards, MD, Kate Agopsowicz, BSc, Theresa L Whiteside, PhD
AltaRex Corp., US Oncology, Dallas, TX; Magee-Women, University of Pittsburgh Cancer Institute, Pittsburgh, PA

Oregovomab (OvaRex® MAb-B43.13) is a murine monoclonal antibody (MAb) studied in multiple clinical trials as adjunctive immunotherapy for epithelial ovarian cancer (EOC). The i.v. administered MAb modulates immunity by complex formation with the circulating tumor-associated antigen CA125 or CA125-expressing tumor cells, followed by uptake of these immune complexes (IC) by antigen-presenting cells (APC) and preferential processing and presentation to T cells. T cell responses are monitored in multiple Phase II trials conducted in patients (pts) with recurrent EOC or after primary therapy pre and post oregovomab administrations. The ELISPOT assay for IFN-gamma was optimized using normal donors and ovarian cancer patients including choice of antigen presenting cells (APC), need and length of in vitro sensitization (IVS) to enrich T cell precursors, titration of the antigen, and incubating the CA125 antigen alone or in complex with the CA125-specific antibody, MAb-B43.13. The optimal conditions were determined to be a 24-h ELISPOT assay with a 7-day IVS step and DC as APC. Most donors and ovarian cancer patients responded best to DC pulsed with CA125 in immune complexed form compared to CA125 alone. Optimum responses were seen using CA125 concentrations of 500 U/mL and 5 µg/mL of MAb-B43.13. Subsequently, clinical trial samples were analyzed in this optimized ELISPOT assay using autologous DC pulsed with either CA125 alone, MAb alone, or CA125-MAb IC, prior to restimulation with autologous tumor, CA125, or MAb for 24 h. oregovomab was well tolerated and induced multiple antigen-specific immune responses. T cell responses were commonly induced after 4 doses and were associated with prolonged time to disease progression and survival in the one completed trial with T cell monitoring to date (Study OVA-Gy-12: $p<0.0001$, and $p=0.008$, respectively, log-rank test). In this study, 7 of 18 (39%) pts demonstrated significant ($p<0.05$) increases over baseline in T cell precursors to CA125 and 5 of 8 (63%) pts to autologous tumor (randomization test). T cell responses were MHC class I and II restricted and were activated more efficiently when the IVS was conducted with IC rather then CA125 or MAb alone, as seen with normal donors. Interestingly, in this combined trial of oregovomab and chemotherapy in recurrent disease pts, T cell responses to autologous tumor increased after completion of chemo-immuno therapy. By targeting CA125 or apoptotic tumor cells to APC (in particular DC) via the oregovomab, the data indicate that clinical administration of low dose murine antibodies, even in the setting of combined treatment with cytotoxic chemotherapy, may act as an efficient and well tolerated immunotherapeutic approach to induce helper and cytotoxic T cells and to improve clinical outcomes.

O-64

CELL TRANSPLANTATION INTO POLYACRYLAMIDE GEL IMPLANTED TO ANIMALS UNDER THE SKIN: LONG-TERM MAINTENANCE OF CELL VIABILITY *IN VIVO* AND POSSIBLE APPLICATIONS IN ONCOLOGY AND ENDOCRINOLOGY

S. E. Severin
Moscow Research Institute of Medical Ecology, Moscow, Russia

Inert gels causing no immunological rejection upon transplantation are widely employed in plastic surgery for correction of various cosmetic defects. After implantation, such gels become enclosed into a connective tissue capsule which creates favorable conditions for the growth and viability of various body cells. Xeno- or allogeneic cells protected from recipient's effector cells by connective tissue capsules produce long-lasting therapeutic or immunizing effects. In this study, xenogeneic human (melanoma SK-MEL-1) and mouse (melanoma B-16) tumor cells retained their viability in polyacrylamide gel injected to rats under the skin up to a period of 3 months. The immunizing effect of xenotransplantation of tumor cells was studied by transplantation of cells of human tumors, melanoma SK-MEL-1 and adenocarcinoma MCF-7 into polyacrylamide gel implanted to C57Black/6 mice under the skin. A significant protective effect was observed after injection of syngeneic tumor cells, melanoma B-16 and adenocarcinoma Ca-755 to mice immunized with human cells. Immunization of animals with xenogeneic tumors was accompanied by the development of cell-mediated cytotoxic responses and an increase in the titers of cross-reacting antibodies in mouse blood sera. The splenocytes of mice immunized with human melanoma cells and stored in polyacrylamide gel over a long period of time were used to obtain a panel of monoclonal antibodies reacting with the antigenic determinants common for mouse and human melanoma. After transplantation of polyacrylamide gel to rats, normal xenogeneic neonatal pancreatic rabbit and piglet cells retained their viability and secreted insulin during at least one month. In rats with experimental streptocytosine diabetes, such transplantation caused reduction of glucose content in the blood sera to a normal level. Allotransplantation of mouse tumor cells into the gel capsules of non-syngeneic BALB/c mice induced the growth of implanted tumors to an extent which markedly exceeded the volume of the implanted gel. There was no rejection of the allogeneic tumor despite its obvious immunological incompatibility with the recipient's organism. This finding suggests that efficient protection from immune mechanisms of recipients with connective tissue capsules can be afforded by therapeutic transplantation of normal allogeneic endocrine cells to patients with diabetes and other pathological conditions. The use of an inert gel able to be encapsulated within animal or human organisms in oncological and endocrinological practice for correction of immunological responses to xeno- and allografts, viz., their enhancement in xenotransplantation of tumor cells or inhibition in allotransplantation of normal cells, seems to be a very promising approach.

O-65

A BISPECIFIC ANTIBODY (BAB) DIRECTED AGAINST CARCINOEMBRYONIC ANTIGEN (CEA) AND TUMOR NECROSIS FACTOR ALPHA (TNFα) TO ENHANCE ANTI-TUMOR EFFECTS OF TNFα COMBINED WITH RADIOTHERAPY (RT) IN HUMAN DIGESTIVE CANCERS

D. Azria, M. Dorvillius, V. Garambois, S. Gourgou, P. Martineau, B. Robert, M. Ychou, J.B. Dubois, A. Pèlegrin
Tumor Immunotargeting and Antibody Engineering, EMI 0227, INSERM, Department of Radiation Oncology Biostatistics, Unit, CNRS UMR 5094, Department of Medical Oncology Val d'Aurelle–Paul Lamarque Cancer Institute, Montpellier, France

Introduction : TNFα enhances x-ray killing of human tumor cells in vitro and enhances tumor control when combined with RT in animal tumor models. In multiple phase I studies, intravenous injections of TNFα appeared to have severe systemic side effects. To overcome these limitations, we used a BAb directed against CEA and human TNFα to target this cytokine in human digestive carcinoma treated with simultaneous radiation therapy. **Materials and Methods:** We used human digestive carcinoma cell lines (colon cancer, LS174T and pancreatic cancer, BxPC3) to determine the interaction of TNFα and radiation on clonogenic cytotoxicity. Isobolograms were established to confirm additive or supra-additive effect between both treatments. LS174T and BxPC3 cells were grafted s.c. at day 0 into nude mice (7-8 weeks old, female). When tumors reached a volume of about 80 mm^3, mice were randomly assigned to treatments: 1) Normal saline i.v. injection for control group; 2) TNFα at 1 µg/i.v. injection; 3) BAb at 25 µg/i.v. injection; 4) BAb + TNFα (ratio 25µg:1µg) i.v. injection; 5) Local radiation + normal saline (0.5 $Gy.min^{-1}$) at a total dose of 30 Gy delivered in 5 fractions; 6) Local radiation + TNFα injections 3 hours before irradiation; 7) Local radiation + BAb + TNFα co-injected 24 hours before RT. Tumor growth delay was used as the endpoint for all groups. **Results:** In vitro, in LS174T experiments, TNFα added 12 hours before RT showed a statistically significant decrease in the survival fraction at 2 Gy as compared with RT alone (0.23 vs 0.42 Gy, p=0.0017). These results were confirmed with the BxPC3 cell line (0.29 vs 0.72, p<0.00001). Isobolograms confirmed additivity between TNFα and radiation therapy in both cell lines. At 50% survival, data points were within the envelope of additivity. Concerning in vivo experiments, in LS174T and BxPC3 xenografts, radiation therapy as a single agent (group 5) slowed tumor progression as compared to group 1 (p<0.001), whereas TNFα, BAb or BAb + TNFα administered alone (groups 2, 3 and 4) had no effect. In LS174T model, TNFα-RT combination enhanced the delay to reach 2000 mm^3 as compared to RT alone but without statistical difference. This delay was significantly longer when BAb was added (p=0.038, for group 6 vs group 7). In BxPC3 experiments, median delays to reach 2000 mm^3 were similar between RT and TNFα-RT groups (93 days). The use of our BAb in combination with TNFα and RT enhanced significantly this median delay (>128 jours, p=0.0014). No body weight loss was observed in any group. **Conclusion:** These results suggest that TNFα in combination with RT may be beneficial for the treatment of locally advanced digestive cancer without morbidity thanks to our BAb.

O-66

DETECTION OF DISSEMINATED TUMOR CELLS IN REGIONAL LYMPH NODES OF COLORECTAL CANCER PATIENTS USING REAL-TIME QUANTITATIVE RT-PCR FOR CARCINOEMBRYONIC ANTIGEN (CEA) MRNA

Sten Hammarström, PhD, Åke Öberg, MD, Anne Israelsson, BMA, Gudrun Lindmark, MD, PhD, Marie-Louise Hammarström, PhD
Departments of Immunology and Surgery, Umeå University; Surgery, Helsinborgs Hospital, Umeå, Sweden

Presence of metastatic lymph nodes in cancer patients is an indicator of poor prognosis, and as such, a selection instrument of patients to additional chemotherapy. The aim of this project was to develop a specific and sensitive method for detection of lymph nodes infested with tumor cells in patients with colorectal cancer thereby allowing early detection of micrometastases. CEA was chosen as marker for disseminated tumor cells since it is selectively expressed in epithelial cells of the large bowel and expression is maintained in colorectal carcinoma. A real-time quantitative RT-PCR assay with RNA copy standard was constructed. It is specific without signals for CEA-gene family members expressed in immune cells. Linearity between number of PCR cycles and log RNA concentration is seen from 10 to 108 copies and 20 CEA mRNA copies admixed in 200 ng RNA from blood mononuclear cells can be detected. Lymph nodes were collected from resected specimens of patients undergoing surgery for colorectal tumors in Dukes' stages A-C (any TN0-1M0; n = 42), a palliative procedure due to distant metastases (Dukes' stage D; n = 9), inflammatory bowel disease (n = 9) and rectal prolapse (n = 1). CEA mRNA levels were determined in RNA extracted from one half of the lymph node and normalized to the content of 18S rRNA. Results were compared to histopathology and anti-CEA immunohistochemistry. CEA levels in preoperative serum were determined by ELISA. CEA mRNA levels were significantly increased in lymph nodes of patients with colorectal carcinoma (Dukes' stages A-D) compared to lymph nodes from patients with non-malignant conditions (P = 0.003 to 0.0005). In cancer patients the CEA mRNA levels varied from 10-3 to 103 copies/18S rRNA unit and the average level in patients with Dukes' stage C was significantly higher than in patients with Dukes' A and B. However, 50% of the patients in the Dukes' B group had CEA mRNA levels within the range of the Dukes' C group. Determination of CEA mRNA in lymph nodes was significantly superior to anti-CEA immunohistochemistry in revealing signs of occult disease. Serum levels of CEA did not correlate to CEA mRNA levels or overt micrometastases in lymph nodes. Whether lymph node micrometastases are associated with clinically relevant metastases in colorectal cancer has not yet been proven, but we have shown that quantitative determination of CEA mRNA in lymph nodes may identify an additional number of patients that possibly may benefit from adjuvant chemotherapy.

O-68

THE ROLE OF VCAM, ICAM, SELECTIN E AND SELECTIN P IN DETECTION OF LIVER METASTASES OF COLORECTAL CARCINOMA

Lubos Holubec Jr., MD, PhD, Ondrej Topolcan, MD, PhD, Prof., Jindrich Finek, MD, Richard Pikner, MD, Ladislav Pecen, MD, Lubos Holubec, MD, PhD, Vladimir Visokai, MD, Ludmila Lipska, MD
Faculty Hospital Pilsen, Academy of Science, Thomayer's Hospital Praque, Czech Republic

Aim of the study: In connection with the metastatic process of colorectal carcinoma into the liver, experimental research attributes a significant role to the activation of adhesive molecules (ICAM, VCAM, E and P selectins) which participate, together with CEA, in the adhesion of metastatic tumor cells and thrombocyte aggregates to the activated endothelium of liver vessels. This pathological process is one of the decisive factors in the formation of secondary liver metastases. The assessment of adhesive molecules, in combination with CEA, therefore seems to be a factor in the early detection of liver metastases in patients with colorectal carcinoma. The aims of the pilot study were to find out the approximate relationship between the levels of adhesive molecules in serum and the levels of tumor marker values. Furthermore in accordance with the results of the pilot study we focused on the optimalization of the programme of longitudinal monitoring of patients with colorectal carcinoma, aiming at early detection of liver metastases.
Methodology: The adhesives molecules ICAM, VCAM, Selectin E and Selectin P (Bender Medsystem) were analyzed in a group of 40 healthy individuals, 40 patients with benign GIT disease and 40 patients with generalization of colorectal tumors into the liver. The results of adhesive molecule assessment were compared with the CEA, CA 19-9, TPS and TPA serum levels. **Results:** In all patients with metastatic liver the VCAM values, and in most cases also ICAM values, were significantly increased. On the other hand, values of Selectin E and Selectin P were increased only in single cases. In cases of metastatic liver we proved a statistically significant correlation between VCAM, ICAM and proliferation tumor markers (TPS, TPA) and also with CEA. **Conclusions:** The result of the pilot study was that the most important of the adhesives molecules is VCAM, followed by ICAM, which undoubtedly play an important role in the metastatic proces of colorectal carcinoma into the liver. The importance of Selectin E and P is limited. We found the best correlation between VCAM and ICAM. These two adhesive molecules also correlate significantly with CEA, cytokeratines and proliferative tumor markers. In addition to CEA, the values for VCAM had the most significant relation to a bad prognosis. This study was supported by the grants: ME CR 13/98: 111400003 and ME 438.

O-69

CHANGES IN CEA SERUM LEVELS DURING FIRST-LINE CHEMOTHERAPY AS A PREDICTOR OF RESPONSE TO THERAPY AND TIME TO PROGRESSION IN PATIENTS WITH ADVANCED COLORECTAL CANCER (ACC)

Marco Tampellini, MD, PhD, Andrea Saini, MD, Maria Pia Brizzi, MD, Gabriella Gorzegno, MD, Emiliano Aroasio, MD, Alfredo Berruti, MD, Raffaella Bitossi, MD, Mirella Torta, MD, Paola Bellati, MD, Luigi Dogliotti, MD, PhD
Oncologia Medica, Dipartiento di Scienze Cliniche e Biologiche, Università degli Studi di Torino; ASO S. Luigi di Orbassano, Abbott, Divisione Diagnostici; Roma, Italy

While sensitivity and specificity of CEA is well known, the role of this marker in monitoring response to therapy and in predicting survival of ACC pts is still controversial. Bimonthly serum determination of CEA with an automated chemiluminescent method Abbott Architect i2000 (Abbott, Abbott Park, Illinois, USA) during therapy is a general common practice in our institution. We then reviewed the clinical records of 103 pts treated from January 2000 to December 2002 with oxaliplatin or irinotecan based chemotherapy as first-line treatment. We extracted CEA levels at the time of first disease relapse before any treatment onset, and at 3 and 6 months during treatment together with the clinical profile of the pts. Patients' characteristics were: median age (range) 59 (29-77); male/female 69/34; colon/rectum 70/33; 1 mts site/>1 mts site 64/39; mts in liver 72/103 (69.9%); lung 28/103 (27.2%); peritoneum 23/103 (22.3%); locally advanced 26/103 (25.2%). At baseline, CEA values >5 U/ml were found in 72/103 pts (overall sensitivity: 69.9%). Abnormal marker values were recorded in 57/72 pts (79.2%) with liver mts, 20/28 pts (71.4%) with lung mts, 16/26 pts (61.5%) with peritoneal mts, 11/23 pts (47.8%) with locally advanced disease, 44/64 pts (68.7%) with 1 mts site, 28/39 pts (71.8%) with >1 mts site; 14/22 pts (63.6%) with primary disease in the right colon, 33/48 pts (68.7%) in left colon, and 25/33 pts (75.7%) in rectum. Clinical responses were evident in 49/103 pts (47.6%), whereas 45/103 pts (43.7%) obtained a disease stabilization and 9/103 pts (8.7%) progressed. Considering only pts with elevated CEA values at baseline, 23/32 responding pts (71.9%) presented a marker reduction >50%, whereas a marker increase >50% was found in 5/8 progressing pts (62.5%). Median times to progression were 14.8 mo for pts with decreasing CEA values and 8.3 mo for those who presented a marker increase (p<0.01). At the time of data computation, 52/103 pts (50.5%) died, with a median overall survival (OS) of 32 mo. Pts with normal CEA levels at baseline survived significantly longer than their counterpart (median OS 40 mo vs 29.4 mo, p<0.001). OSs according to marker changes were: 29 mo for pts with a decrease >50% and 15 mo for pts with a >50% marker increase (p<0.01). These preliminary results demonstrated that serum CEA variations are strongly correlated to the response to therapy and to the TTP, representing a good predictor of OS. Data collection is still ongoing and updated results will be presented.

O-70

THE ROLE OF CA 19-9 AS A PREDICTOR OF SURVIVAL OF PATIENTS WITH NEWLY DIAGNOSED ADVANCED COLORECTAL CANCER (ACC)

Andrea Saini, MD, Marco Tampellini, MD, PhD, Maria Pia Brizzi, MD, Gabriella Gorzegno, MD, Emiliano Aroasio, MD, Alfredo Berruti, MD, Raffaella Bitossi, MD, Mirella Torta, MD, Paola Bellati, MD, Luigi Dogliotti, MD, PhD
Oncologia Medica, Dipartimento di Scienze Cliniche e Biologiche, Università degli Studi di Torino; ASO S. Luigi di Orbassano, Abbott, Divisione Diagnostici; Roma, Italy

In the last few years, the introduction of Oxaliplatin and Irinotecan in the treatment of pts with ACC permitted to obtain an important increase in overall survival (OS). However, some pts does not benefit from these new drugs and presents a progressive disease. An easy-available, low-cost test that allow physicians to predict survival outcome is then a much-needed clinical tool. We reviewed the clinical records of 103 pts treated and followed from January 2000 to December 2001 by our Institution in which CA 19-9 levels were determined through an automated chemiluminescent method Abbott Architect i2000 (Abbott, Abbott Park, Illinois, USA) at three time points: baseline at the time of first disease relapse before any treatment onset, at 3 and 6 months during first-line treatment. Patients' characteristics were: median age (range) 59 (29-77); male/female 69/34; colon/rectum 70/33; 1 mts site/>1 mts site 64/39; mts in liver 72/103 (69.9%); lung 28/103 (27.2%); peritoneum 23/103 (22.3%); locally advanced 26/103 (25.2%). At baseline, CA 19-9 values >37 U/ml were found in 47/103 pts (overall sensitivity: 45.6%). Abnormal marker values were recorded in 38/72 pts (52.8%) with liver mts, 11/28 pts (39.3%) with lung mts, 13/26 pts (50%) with peritoneal mts, 9/23 pts (39.1%) with locally advanced disease, 25/64 pts (39.1%) with 1 mts site, and 22/39 pts (56.4%) with >1 mts site. Clinical responses were evident in 49/103 pts (47.6%), whereas 45/103 pts (43.7%) obtained a disease stabilization and 9/103 pts (8.7%) progressed. At the time of data computation, 52/103 pts (50.5%) died, with a median OS of 32 mo. Pts with normal CA 19-9 levels at baseline survived significantly longer than their counterpart (median OS 42 mo vs 23 mo, p<0.001). OSs according to marker changes were: 45 mo for pts with normal CA 19-9 values at baseline that remained unchanged during therapy, 23 mo for pts with a decrease >50% and 17 mo for pts with a >50% marker increase (p<0.01). In the multivariate Cox analysis, only changes in CA 19-9 levels were an independent variable for OS. These preliminary results demonstrated that CA 19-9 is an easy-available predictive parameter for survival that permitted to discriminate those pts with an aggressive disease from those with a more indolent form. Data collection is ongoing and updated results will be presented.

O-71

CLINICOPATHOLOGIC AND PROGNOSTIC SIGNIFICANCE OF MATRILYSIN EXPRESSION AT THE INVASIVE FRONT IN HUMAN COLORECTAL CANCERS

Fumio Itoh, MD, PhD, Hiroyuki Yamamoto, MD, PhD, Yasushi Adachi, MD, PhD, Shina Horiuchi, Mio Yoshida, Katsuhiko Nosho, Hiroaki Taniguchi, Yongfen Min, MD, PhD, Akravit Vinitketkumnuen, Kohzoh Imai, MD, PhD
Sapporo Medical University, Sapporo, Japan

Matrix metalloproteinases have been implicated in tumor progression. Matrilysin, one of the matrix metalloproteinases, is frequently overexpressed in gastrointestinal cancers. The aim of our study was to assess the validity of matrilysin as a prognostic marker of colorectal cancers. Matrilysin expression was immunohistochemically analyzed using formalin-fixed, paraffin-embedded specimens from 113 colorectal cancer patients who had undergone curative surgery. The lumenal surface of neoplastic glands in the superficial layer was apically stained, while the cytoplasm of cancer cells at the invasive front was diffusely stained for matrilysin. Sections with immunostaining signals in more than 30% of carcinoma cells at the invasive front, which were observed in 47 (42%) cases, were judged as being positive for matrilysin. Matrilysin positivity was significantly correlated with the depth of invasion, lymph node metastasis, lymphatic invasion, advanced Dukes' stage, and poor outcome. Patients with matrilysin-positive cancer had a significantly shorter overall survival time than those with matrilysin-negative cancer. For patients with intermediate invasive tumor (T2 or T3), only matrilysin was a significant prognostic variable for predicting overall survival in multivariate analysis. Matrilysin expression at the invasive front could be an important marker, predicting an unfavorable prognosis after surgical treatment in patients with colorectal cancer. It is well known that matrilysin is effectively activated by matrix serine protease trypsin. We will also present the results showing that patients with concomitant overexpression of matrilysin and trypsin at the invasive front, in which they were often colocalized, had the worst prognosis.

O-72

CATHEPSIN B AND MATRIX METALLOPROTEINASE-9 IN COLORECTAL CANCERS: SINGLE MARKER VS. DOUBLE MARKER PROFILES

Mary Murnane, PhD, Jinguo Cai, Sania Shuja, PhD, MD, Kwonseop Kim, PhD, Christine Iacobuzio-Donahue, PhD
Boston University School of Medicine, Boston, MA; University of Florida Health Science Center, Jacksonville, FL; Chonnam University, S Korea; Johns Hopkins University Medical Center, Baltimore, MD

Detailed proteomic or genomic characterizations of cancer/normal tissue pairs provides a new approach to subtyping cancers that may permit 'fine-tuning' of cancer prognoses for optimal assignment of patients to treatment protocols. In our studies, we have analyzed more than 250 patient-matched normal and colorectal cancer tissues for a double marker profile of cathepsin B (CatB) and matrix metalloproteinase-9 (MMP-9), with both enzymes assayed in the identical tissue extracts. Tissues were snap-frozen immediately after surgery and stored at -80oC prior to extraction. All extracts were assayed for total soluble protein and enzyme specific activities, using a highly specific substrate (Z-Ala-Arg-Arg-MNA) for CatB and gelatin zymography with computerized band assessment for MMP-9. Additional characterization was obtained by assaying for CatL, CatH and MMP-2 activities, K-ras mutations and p53 LOH. Resulting data indicate that CatB and MMP-9 activities were inversely expressed in the majority of cancers, with CatB levels high when MMP-9 levels were low and vice versa. This inverse expression pattern was not observed for other proteolytic markers analyzed in the same extracts. Analyses of a large set of colorectal cancers identified 4 CatB/MMP-9 activity profiles, including two profiles seen in the majority of cases: either(1) high CatB with low MMP-9 activities or (2)low CatB with high MMP-9 activities; and two profiles seen in a smaller number of cases: either (3) high CatB with high MMP-9 or (4) low CatB with low MMP-9 activities. Patient survival data on these cases are now being analyzed using a set of Cox proportional hazards models to test the extent to which either CatB or MMP-9 as individual markers versus the 4 CatB/MMP-9 double marker profiles can predict the risk of death among colorectal cancer patients at all stages.

O-73

UPA AND UPA:PAI-1 COMPLEXES IN SERUM AND PLASMA

David E. Jarosz, MS, Leticia D. Morris, BS, William J. Tighe, Siobhan B. Walsh, Dhaval R. Trivedi, Walter P. Carney, PhD, Peter J. Hamer, MA
Oncogene Science/Bayer Diagnostics, Cambridge, MA

A number of proteases allow the passage of cells through the basement membrane and into the general circulation. Some of these proteases have been studied as markers of metastasis, since they are instrumental in allowing the extravasation and intravasation of tumor cells. Our studies have centered on the plasminogen activation (PA) system, specifically the markers urokinase-type plasminogen activator (uPA) and complexes of uPA with its inhibitor, plasminogen activator inhibitor type 1 (PAI-1). The formation of uPA:PAI-1 Complexes only occurs if uPA and PAI-1 are in their active form. In addition, while serum is a viable matrix for the uPA ELISA, plasma is the sample of choice for the uPA:PAI-1 Complex ELISA. This is due to the large amount of PAI-1 contained in platelets that is released when the clotting process occurs. We have developed commercially available ELISA assays for the detection and quantitation of uPA and uPA:PAI-1 complexes in human plasma samples. In order to establish a normal range for uPA and uPA:PAI-1 Complexes, normal serum (uPA) and normal plasma (uPA:PAI-1 Complexes) were analyzed by ELISA. For uPA 118 normal sera were tested and the mean value obtained was 1192 pg/mL. The normal range (mean +/- two standard deviations) was 459 - 1924 pg/mL. For uPA:PAI-1 Complexes the normal mean value was 115 pg/mL with the upper limit of normal of 293 pg/mL. Once a normal range was established for each marker, serum and plasma samples from a variety of cancer patients were analyzed. The uPA levels were elevated in colon and pancreatic cancer. With uPA:PAI-1 Complexes, elevations were seen in a number of cancer types. Specifically, 52% of the breast cancers, 16% of the colon cancers, 16% of the lung cancer and 20% of the prostate cancer samples had uPA:PAI-1 Complex levels above the normal cutoff. This type of data may prove important for selecting and/or monitoring patients receiving therapies directed to components of the plasminogen activation system.

O-74

CANCER ANTIGEN ASSOCIATED SERPIN (CASERPIN) FORMS STABLE COMPLEXES WITH CA125, MUC1 AND PSA IN SERUM

Yuri S. Lebedin, MD, Sergey V. Chukanov, MD, Sergey A. Prokofiev, MD, Maya A. Zhdanovich, MD, Andrey Y. Toptygin, MD
Xema-Medica Co Ltd, Moscow, Russia

Caserpin is a neoantigen generated in serum alpha-1-protease inhibitor (alpha-1-antitrypsin) after specific binding to trypsin like proteases. Caserpin neoantigen contains at least two distinct epitopes recognized by monoclonal antibodies. In freshly drawn normal serum or plasma the contents of caserpin detected by ELISA is lower than 10 ng/ml.

Affinity purified caserpin was isolated from normal spleen extract and two tumor materials - a pleuritic fluid from lung carcinoma patient and an ascitic fluid from ovarian carcinoma patient. All three purified preparations have shown high homology to alpha-1-protease inhibitor in mass spectrometry (MALDI-TOF), and strongly reacted to commercial rabbit antiserum against alpha-1-antitrypsin. In SDS-PAGE, caserpin preparations were located between 40 and 60 kDa depending on source material.

Surprisingly, caserpin antigen was detected in HMW mucin fraction of tumor ascitic fluids and tissue extracts. In two site ELISAs constructed from anti-caserpin mAbs as a capture, we have detected hetero-complexes with mAbs to CA125 antigen, MUC1 (peptide repeat); total and free PSA in sera of cancer patients. In some cases, the hetero-complexes of caserpin with CA125, MUC1 and PSA were clearly detected in absence of detectable "regular" tumor marker antigens. The biological role of free caserpin and the mechanism of interaction between caserpin antigen and tumor marker antigens are unclear. However, we concluded that the revealed neoantigen is able to form stable complexes with known tumor markers and to interfere with the existing methods of their detection.

O-75

GM-CSF BASED CANCER VACCINES

Glenn Dranoff, MD
Dana-Farber Cancer Institute, Boston, MA

We have demonstrated that vaccination with irradiated tumor cells engineered to secrete granulocyte-macrophage colony stimulating factor (GM-CSF) stimulates potent, specific, and long lasting anti-tumor immunity in multiple murine tumor model systems. Vaccination requires the participation of CD4 and CD8 positive T lymphocytes, CD1d restricted NKT cells, and high titer IgG antibodies and likely involves improved tumor antigen presentation by recruited dendritic cells and macrophages. Clinical testing of GM-CSF based tumor cell vaccines has revealed that many of the principles derived from murine studies are relevant to patients with advanced cancer. Metastatic melanoma patients injected with lethally irradiated, autologous tumor cells engineered by retroviral mediated gene transfer to secrete GM-CSF consistently develop brisk infiltrates of dendritic cells expressing high levels of B7-1 at vaccination sites. These reactions initiate the generation of systemic immunity characterized by the dense infiltration of distant metastases with CD4 and CD8 positive T lymphocytes and plasma cells which effectuate extensive tumor destruction (at least 80%), fibrosis, and edema in approximately two-thirds of treated patients. Anti-melanoma cytotoxic and helper T cell and IgG antibody responses are associated with tumor destruction. In an effort to expand this vaccination strategy to tumor types not amenable to short-term culture, we have been exploring the use of adenoviral mediated gene transfer to engineer autologous tumor cells to secrete GM-CSF. In this scheme, metastatic lesions are processed to single cell suspension by mechanical and enzymatic digestion; tumor cells are then infected overnight with an E1, E3 deleted adenoviral vector expressing GM-CSF, irradiated, and cryopreserved. Phase I clinical trials of this approach are underway for patients with metastatic nonsmall cell lung carcinoma, metastatic ovarian carcinoma, metastatic melanoma, and advanced myelodysplasia/acute myelogenous leukemia.

O-76

SERIAL ANALYSIS OF CIRCULATING TUMOR CELLS (CTC'S) BY CK19 MRNA EXPRESSION AND SHED HER-2 EXTRACELLULAR DOMAIN IN HER-2 POSITIVE METASTATIC BREAST CANCER PATIENTS TREATED WITH Anti-HER-2 (HERCEPTIN) THERAPY

Lyndsay Harris, Raquel Nunes ,Taylor Ngo, Mamta Gakhar, Julia Keller, Lisa Roberts, Harold Burstein, Eric Winer, J. Dirk Iglehart, Paula Freidman
Dana-Farber Cancer Institute, Boston, MA; Abbott Laboratories, Abbott Park, IL

Purpose: To evaluate the feasibility of detecting CTCs by CK19 mRNA in patients with HER-2 positive metastatic breast cancer and correlate this with serum HER-2 and clinical response to Herceptin therapy. **Patients and Methods:** Blood samples were collected from 55 women with HER-2 positive (IHC+++ and/or FISH+) metastatic breast cancer and 30 healthy female volunteers. Blood samples were collected at baseline, during with the first cycle of H&N at weeks 2, 3 and 5, and at each restaging. Peripheral blood mononuclear cells were isolated and enriched for epithelial cells by immunomagnetic selection (DynabeadsÒ). Plasma was used to measure shed HER-2 extracellular domain using as commerically available kit (HER-2/neu ELISAÒ; Oncogene Science) The presence of CK19 gene mRNA was determined by RT-PCR using the LCx probe system (Abbott Laboratories). Thirty healthy donor blood samples were accessed as controls. **Results:** A total of 158 samples, from 24 patients were analyzed. Samples at baseline and first restaging were available in 22 patients, of which 10 had CK19 detectable (45%). CTC were only detected in patients with liver metastases (p=0.0004). All patients with CK 19 present at baseline responded to therapy. In subsequent cycles CK 19 remained negative in most patients. In two cases, low positive values were detectable prior to clinical progression. CK-19 mRNA was undetectable in 29/30 (97%) of healthy controls. In this study, 48/55 patients had serial samples available for analysis of shed HER-2. Of these, 21/48 (44%) had elevated ECD using a cut-off value of 20 ng/ml. Serum HER2 was correlated with both disease burden and visceral disease (p=0.018) and the percentage change was associated with disease progression. The comparison of serum HER-2 and CK-19 from the same patient show consistent expression patterns of shed HER-2 and CK-19. **Conclusions:** Results of this study suggest that CTCs are detectable by RT-PCR for CK-19 and that this may identify a group of patients with metastatic liver disease. The pattern of CTC detection mirrors that of circulating HER-2 and that their behavior is consistent with clinical response to Herceptin therapy. A validation dataset will be presented.

P-1

MONITORING SERUM HER-2/NEU ONCOPROTEIN LEVELS IN METASTATIC BREAST CANCER PATIENTS

Sheryl Brown-Shimer, BS, Karen Johnson, BS, Walter Carney, PhD
Oncogene Science/Bayer Diagnostics, Cambridge, MA

HER-2/neu is a membrane bound growth factor receptor, and the extracellular domain (ECD) is shed from the surface of cancer cells. The HER-2 ECD, quantified in serum using an ELISA, has been shown to be shed into the blood of normal individuals and can be found at elevated levels in women with metastatic breast cancer (MBC). A retrospective study of patients on various therapeutic regimens was performed to evaluate the clinical utility of the Oncogene Science/Bayer Diagnostics HER-2/neu Microtiter ELISA in monitoring and management of patients with MBC. The Upper Limit of Normal was determined to be 15 ng/ml HER-2/neu, patients with serum levels above this number are considered to be elevated. In order to monitor patients, a normal longitudinal variability was established from 38 normal patients monitored monthly for 6 months to be less than 20%. MBC patients with initial (pre-treatment) serum Her-2/neu values of 15 ng/ml or above were monitored by ELISA. The longitudinal changes in their serum HER-2/neu values over time were compared to the clinical course of their disease established by clinical tests at each visit during treatment. Serial increases in HER-2/neu were reflective of progressive disease, while decreasing serum HER-2/neu was reflective of response to therapy. Since the HER-2/neu Oncoprotein has also become an important therapeutic target for treating women with MBC, continuous assessment of patient serum HER-2/neu status during MBC is an important tool in the treatment and management of these women. The anti-HER-2 monoclonal antibody (Herceptin®) therapy, does not interfere in the serum HER-2/neu ELISA. Concordance of longitudinal HER-2/neu changes to clinical course of disease was observed when monitoring MBC patients on monoclonal antibody therapy, as it was for MBC patients on other therapies. Our studies demonstrate that monitoring serum HER-2/neu ECD levels during MBC may be an important test for managing the treatment of MBC patients with HER-2/neu positive tumors.

P-2

COMPARISON OF SERUM, EDTA-PLASMA AND HEPARIN-PLASMA RESULTS FOR THE ABBOTT FREE PSA AND TOTAL PSA ASSAYS*

Barry Dowell, Shin Egawa, Kimberlee Borden
Abbott Laboratories, Abbott Park, IL; Kitasato University, Tokyo, Japan; Research Oriented Biostatistics, Inc., Mundelein, IL

Serum PSA is the most useful tumor marker for the management and early detection of prostate cancer. The Abbott AxSYM® Free and Total PSA assays are designed to quantitate PSA in serum; however, recent reports have shown that free PSA is more stable in plasma than in serum. Two independent studies were performed to compare the performance of the Abbott PSA assays using serum and plasma. In the first study, serum and EDTA-plasma samples from 344 men who underwent prostate biopsy with total PSA values <50 ng/mL were evaluated by linear regression using the Abbott assays. For the Abbott Total PSA assay, plasma total PSA = 0.934 X serum total PSA + 0.077 with r = 0.997. The results for the Abbott Free PSA assay were: plasma Free PSA = 0.9996 X serum free PSA + 0.008 with r = 0.997. For % Free PSA, the results were: plasma % Free PSA = 1.021 X serum % Free PSA + 0.008, r = 0.988). In this patient cohort, serum performed slightly better than plasma for the early detection of prostate cancer (Egawa et al. J. Urology 167:97-102, 2002). In the second study, purified PSA at two levels was added to serum, EDTA-plasma and heparin-plasma from 40 healthy male volunteers (20 for each PSA level). Free PSA and total PSA levels were determined and the results for plasma were compared to those for serum as a percentage. For the low and high levels of free PSA, the mean for EDTA-plasma was 98.2% and 98.4%, respectively. For heparin-plasma, the mean for the low and high levels of free PSA was 98.6% and 98.5%, respectively. For the low and high levels of total PSA, the mean for EDTA-plasma was 96.2% and 96.8%, respectively. For heparin-plasma, the mean for the low and high levels of total PSA was 98.4% and 98.5%, respectively. These studies provide an initial comparison of the performance of the Abbott Free and Total PSA assays with serum versus plasma samples and demonstrate comparable results.

*Pending FDA approval

P-3

INS316 (URIDINE 5'-TRIPHOSPHATE, UTP) ENHANCES SPUTUM QUALITY FOR THE DETECTION OF P16 METHYLATION IN LUNG CANCER PATIENTS

Jeanne Harvey, PhD, Allison Gannon, Fred Johnson, PhD, John Lechner, PhD
Bayer Diagnostics, Berkeley, CA; Inspire Pharmaceuticals, Durham, NC

The p16 tumor-suppressor protein is frequently absent in non-small cell lung cancer, and DNA methylation of CpG islands within the promoter has been associated with this loss of gene function. We evaluated a novel agent for sputum induction with regard to its ability to enhance sample collection for detection of p16 promoter methylation using methylation-specific PCR (MSP). INS316 is a P2Y2 receptor agonist that increases airway hydration, cilia beat frequency, mucociliary clearance, and sputum expectoration. Samples were collected in a double-blind crossover, placebo-controlled study testing a single dose effect of INS316 in lung cancer patients prior to surgery. In 19 patient sets, the INS316-induced sputum contained more pulmonary macrophages than placebo (272.8 vs. 159.3) or spontaneous collections (272.8 vs. 43.5). All samples with adequate DNA for MSP analysis should have detectable unmethylated p16 sequences, reflecting the background of DNA from non-cancerous cells in the sputum. 100% of the samples from INS316 dosed patients had detectable amplicon. Yet, only 85% of the samples from patients without INS316 induction yielded amplicon. Methylated sequences in the p16 promoter region were detected in four of the patients. All of these tumors were located in the periphery of the lung. In two of these cases, methylated amplicons were detected only in the INS316-induced samples. INS316 provides an improvement over currently established sputum-induction techniques, especially for sampling cells from peripherally located tumors.

P-4

CHECKING THE COURSE OF COLO-RECTAL CARCINOMA FOLLOW UP USING MATHEMATICAL CLASSIFICATION OF TUMOR MARKER PROFILES

Lubos Holubec Jr. MD, PhD, Norman Botterlich, PhD, Ondrej Topolcan, MD, PhD, Prof, Jindrich Finek, MD, Richard Pikner, MD, Ladislav Pecen, MD, PhD, Lubos Holubec, MD, PhD
Faculty Hospital Pilsen, Czech Republic, pe Diagnostik, Academy of Science, Czech Republic

Introduction: The authors are concerned with a feasibility study using retrospective data of 455 patients with colorectal carcinoma in order to check the course of colo-rectal carcinoma follow-up using mathematical classification of tumor marker profiles. Data are derived from patients‘ records of routine clinical practice during follow-up care of patients (up to 7 years) after primary operation. Therefore the data acquired are characteristic of daily routine practice. **Material and Methods:** Serum levels of CEA (IRMA Immunotech), CA 19-9 and CA 72-4 (IRMA Cis Bio International France) were determined during the follow-up in a group of 455 patients with clinically diagnosed and histologically verified colorectal carcinoma. The results were compared with the retrospectively confirmed clinical status of the patients. Statistical evaluation was performed with the STATISTICA software product (StatSoft Inc.) and by the use of company software of the Pe Diagnostik comp. **Results:** Tumor marker measurement values of clinical status NED and RD show a highly significant ($p< 0,01$) contrast to one another for CEA, CA 19-9 and CA 72-4. However, the sensitivities of single markers are insufficient for a diagnostic decision. As exemplified by CEA it is obvious that the clinical status RD is not always followed by an increase in value of the tumor marker. Above 20% of measurement values of patients with clinical status RD lie below the basis value of 2.3 ng/ml, and differentiation in this zone is not possible. On the other hand in the zone above the basis value of 2.3 ng/ml the sensitivity increases significantly. It is also possible to find such basis values with CA 72-4 (2.2 U/ml) and CA 19-9 (15.0 U/ml. All the RD-measurement values for particular single marker are always below 80% of these basis values, but 95% of the RD measurement values show an increased value in the marker profile at least in one marker. For that reason, the two- and three-parameter classification models are used to assign the clinical status NED, only if all the parameters for the particular threshold value are not exceeded. In this case the clinical status RD is assigned. **Conclusion:** These analyses confirm the thesis that through the evaluation of tumor marker profiles consisting of CEA, CA 19-9 and CA 72-4 , the sensitivity in comparison to the best single marker (CEA) can be increased. This increase is also reasonable, because the single marker often does not exceed the basis zone even if the clinical status RD is proved. However, infrequently with the clinical status RD all markers in the profile yield a conspicuous measurement values. In our analysis we take into account only the absolute measurement values. Furthermore an optimal development would be to analyze whether the inclusion of changes of measurement values during follow-up can also improve sensitivity. This study was supported by the grants: ME CR 13/98: 111400003 and ME 438.

P-5

TENASCIN-C EXPRESSION AND PROGNOSIS IN PANCREATIC CANCER

Anne Juuti, MD, Stig Nordling, MD, PhD, Johanna Louhimo, MD, Johan Lundin, MD, PhD, Caj Haglund, MD, PhD
Department of Surgery, Helsinki University Central Hospital; Department of Pathology, University of Helsinki, Helsinki, Finland

Cancer of the pancreas is a fairly common disease in the Western world. It is associated with an extremely poor outcome. It would be valuable to find prognostic markers to define the patient group that would benefit most from heavy surgical and oncological treatments. Tenascin-C is a potential prognostic marker, recently studied in different malignancies. Tenascin is a large hexameric extracellular matrix protein that is present during embryonic development but essentially absent in normal adult tissue. It is involved in proliferative processes such as wound healing and tumor development. The tissue expression of tenascin-C has been shown to correlate with prognosis in colon cancer, carcinoma of papilla Vater and breast cancer.

In this retrospective study we studied the immunohistochemical expression of tenascin- C in 146 pancreatic adenocarcinomas. Formalin-fixed, paraffin embedded specimens were stained with anti-tenascin-C monoclonal antibodies using the ABC technique. Tenascin-C immunoreactivity was observed in most of the pancreatic carcinoma samples: in only 12 (8.2%) of the samples no stain was seen, in 72 (49.3%) samples it was faint, in 52 (35.6%) moderate and in 10 (6.8%) strong. There was no correlation to patients survival, TNM stage, histological grade, tumor size, tumor location, curativity, age nor gender in our study.

In conclusion: Tenascin-C is expressed in most of the pancreatic carcinoma samples, but in contrary to the results in other cancer forms, it seems not to be a prognostic factor in pancreatic cancer.

P-6

PERFORMANCE OF ABBOTT FREE PSA* ASSAY WITH RESPECT TO THE WHO FREE PSA STANDARD

A. L. Lunceford, BS, M. K. Michalski, BS, K. Rodriguez, PhD, R. Olson, MS, R. Phillips, PhD
Abbott Laboratories, Abbott Park, IL

Prostate specific antigen (PSA) is primarily found in two forms in serum. The most abundant form is PSA-ACT, which is PSA complexed to alpha-1-antichymotrypsin. The other form is uncomplexed, or free PSA. The determination of the percent free PSA value, defined as free PSA divided by total immunodetectable PSA multiplied by 100, has been suggested as a means to help discriminate between benign prostatic hyperplasia (BPH) and prostate cancer. Multiple assays have been developed to measure free PSA, but there has been no assay standardization to a common reference material. The Abbott AxSYM® Free PSA* assay marketed by Abbott Laboratories outside of the U.S. uses calibrators referenced against the Stanford 90:10 PSA Reference Material (96/670) composed of 90% PSA-ACT and 10% free PSA, which the World Health Organization (WHO) adopted as the standard for total PSA assays. WHO accepted a Free PSA standard subsequent to the development of the Free PSA assay. The accuracy of the Abbott Free PSA* assay when reading this WHO Free PSA standard (96/668), composed of 100% free PSA, has not been determined previously. The lyophilized WHO Free PSA standard was reconstituted gravimetrically with deionized water to a concentration of 500 ng/mL. Serial dilutions of the WHO Free PSA standard were then prepared in the same diluent used to prepare the current Abbott Free PSA calibrators. Six dilutions were selected to be run on the Abbott Free PSA assay: 0.244 ng/mL, 0.488 ng/mL, 0.977 ng/mL, 1.95 ng/mL, 3.91 ng/mL, and 7.81 ng/mL. The calculated concentrations of the selected dilutions fell within the dynamic range of the Abbott Free PSA assay (0-10 ng/mL). The percent recovery of each of the dilutions of the WHO Free PSA standard was determined, and the calculated percent recoveries ranged from 92% to 96% with a mean percent recovery of 94%. Recovery of the diluted WHO Free PSA standard was slightly better at the lower end of the dynamic range of the Abbott Free PSA assay than at the higher end. The Abbott Free PSA Assay reads the WHO Free PSA standard (96/668) with accuracy.

* Pending FDA approval

P-7

STABILITY OF FREE PSA IN SERUM AS MEASURED BY THE ABBOTT FREE PSA* ASSAY

A. L. Lunceford, BS, R. Phillips, PhD, R. Olson, MS, K. Rodriguez, PhD
Abbott Laboratories, Abbott Park, IL

Free PSA is a form of prostate specific antigen (PSA) that is useful in the discrimination of prostate cancer from benign prostatic hyperplasia. Abbott Laboratories markets a free PSA assay used to determine serum levels of this antigen. In order to make accurate measurements of serum concentrations of free PSA, the stability of this protein must be known so that the assay is performed within a time frame in which there is minimal fluctuation in free PSA concentration determinations. Whole blood samples were collected from nine patients with free PSA serum concentrations of 0.35 to 7.29 ng/mL. After the serum was separated from the clot, each sample was measured on the Abbott AxSYM® Free PSA* assay to determine a baseline value. The remainder of the serum was divided into aliquots, which were either stored at 2 to 8°C or room temperature. Additional aliquots were subjected to three freeze/thaw cycles. Results show that serum samples stored at 2 to 8°C for one day had an average decrease in free PSA concentration of 5.9% while those samples stored at room temperature for one day experienced an average drop in free PSA concentration of 9.2%. When the storage time was extended to 2 days, the samples stored at 2 to 8°C had an average decrease in free PSA concentration of 8.4%, and the samples stored at room temperature dropped an average of 11.1% in free PSA concentration. There was no significant decrease in free PSA values when the serum samples experienced three freeze/thaw cycles. These samples had a mean percent recovery of 99.1%. Optimally, free PSA specimens should be assayed immediately. If conditions do not permit, serum may be stored for one day at 2 to 8°C before being tested. Specimens must be frozen if they are not to be tested within one day.

* Pending FDA approval

P-8

EXPOSED PEPTIDE IN TAFP YIELDS POTENTIALLY IMPROVED TUMOR MARKER

Gerald J. Mizejewski, PhD, Michael M. Muehlemann, MS
Serometrix LLC, E. Syracuse, NY

Human alpha-fetoprotein (HAFP), a tumor-associated fetal protein, is normally a growth-promoting molecule in its compactly folded native form. However, HAFP contains a growth inhibitory peptide (GIP) motif which lies buried in a molecular cleft. Exposure of the GIP segment can be induced by a conformational change in HAFP following stress/shock stimulation and mild denaturalization, defined as transformed alpha-fetoprotein (tAFP). The GIP has been synthesized, purified, and characterized revealing a beta-sheet/turn secondary structure that elicits molecular interactions, aggregation, and oligomerization. Such properties can endow peptide with the capability to bind to cell surface receptors, hence affecting signal transduction.

As a diagnostic agent, preliminary results suggest that a variety of tumors produce tAFP, a previously undetectable form of AFP that can now be detected via immunoassays designed to target the GIP. Measuring tAFP, and the ratio of tAFP/AFP, potentially provides a much improved cancer diagnostic for the detection of many forms of AFP secreting tumors, particularly in the case of breast tumors and liver carcinomas.

P-9

CHARACTERIZATION OF THE HUMAN AFP RECEPTOR (RECAF) I: RECAF IS A FAMILY OF PROTEINS EXHIBITING AGGREGATION IN CELL EXTRACTS

R. Moro, X. Hu, G. Shen, V. Calvo, A. Kummer
Pacific Biosciences Research Centre, Vancouver, Canada

Alpha-fetoprotein (AFP) is incorporated into fetal and cancer cells via a receptor (RECAF). The molecular weight of RECAF varies from one report to another. Reported values are 250 kDa, 62-67 kDa, 50 kDa, 31 and 18 kDa. In an attempt to clarify the value disparity, we analyzed the molecular weight of RECAF from cancer cell lines by PAGE and gel filtration. To detect RECAF, we used biotin or peroxidase labeled AFP in a binding assay on extracts/ fractions coated plates or in Westerns. Normal peripheral leukocytes used as negative controls showed no AFP binding.

Results:
1) Over 80% competition is obtained with a 100X cold AFP. No competition was found with cold human serum albumin.
2) RECAF is not a single protein, but rather a family consisting of at least 5 members with MW of approximately 62, 50, 40, 31 and 18 kDa. Some of these bands appear as doublets. No bands were observed at higher molecular weights.
3) The 31 and 18 kDa bands are only found in the cell extract pellets (16,000 g) and they require 0.5% SDS to be extracted.
4) The 62, 50 and 40 kDa bands are predominantly found in the supernatants of cell extracts prepared in the absence of SDS. They form high molecular weight aggregates, which are dissociated by SDS.
5) Reducing conditions do not affect the mobility of the bands. Furthermore, the reaction between these bands and labeled AFP is not impaired by the presence of reducing agents such as 2ME in the reaction buffer.

P-10

CHARACTERIZATION OF THE HUMAN AFP RECEPTOR (RECAF) II: THE AFP BINDING SITE OF AFP ON RECAF IS AN N-GLYCAN

R. Moro, G. Song, F. Lakhani
Pacific Biosciences Research Centre, Vancouver, Canada

The receptor for AFP (RECAF), a pan-tumoral oncofetal antigen, consists of a family of proteins exhibiting a wide range of molecular weights. Their reaction to biotinylated AFP (B-AFP) can be evidenced in a binding assay by incubating labeled AFP in ELISA plate wells coated with cancer cell extracts. The binding is specific since a high percentage of competition can be achieved by adding an excess of cold AFP. Treatment of the coated wells with periodate (1-100 mM) results in a decrease of binding activity (up to 90% inhibition) and which is proportional to the periodate concentration. Wells coated with human albumin and treated in identical conditions showed no decrease in binding to a polyclonal anti-HSA antibody after identical periodate treatment, thus strongly suggesting that the AFP binding site on RECAF is a glycan.

To demonstrate that the RECAF peptidic chain is not involved, we designed a competitive assay, in which B-AFP and a cell extract containing RECAF were mixed together and then added to wells coated with the same extract. The higher the concentration of cell extract in solution, the lower the reaction of B-AFP to the RECAF on the plate. Subjecting the cell extract to pepsin digestion for 24 hours at 37°C resulted in no discernible bands by PAGE analysis. The inhibition curve obtained with the digested extracts was identical to that of non-digested extracts, thus indicating that the RECAF binding site is a glycan. Finally, cell extracts incubated in the presence of Tunicamycin, which inhibits N-glycosylation showed a significant decrease in AFP binding. Treating cells with Galactosamide, which inhibits the linking of O-glycans, resulted in no change in binding.

All of these results support the conclusion that AFP binds to an N-glycan on RECAF. Since the latter is a family of proteins, these results suggest that a common glycan with AFP binding activity is attached to several proteins with different functional roles.

P-11

DIFFERENTIATION OF THE CANCER AND NORMAL BLOOD SERA SAMPLES WITH THE RECEPTOR FOR ALPHA-FETOPROTEIN RECAF

Janneta Gulyaeva-Tcherkassova, Ricardo Moro
Pacific Biosciences Research Centre, British Columbia, Canada

The receptor for Alpha-fetoprotein (**RECAF)** was discovered and isolated from embryonic tissues and a variety of malignant tissues and cancer cell lines. The molecular weight of the receptor is controversial. Periodate oxidation and pepsin digestion of the protein showed that RECAF is a glycan, which is highly expressed on malignant cells.

We have developed a competitive Solid Phase Radio-Immunoassay (SPRIA) in which serum RECAF and ^{125}I-labeled **RECAF** compete for binding to a rabbit anti-RECAF polyclonal antibody coating 96-well plates. One hundred and twenty four serum samples were studied (84 normal sera and 40 cancer sera including cervix, breast, head and neck, ovarian, colon cancer, rectal adenocarcinoma, and stomach carcinomas).

Results:

	Mean	SD	n	t	p	d.f.
Normal Sera	810.29	249.12	84	19.57	0.0005	112
CANCER SERA	221.35	81.64	40			

Setting cutoff values is difficult since the distribution of both the cancer and the normal serum populations are skewed toward lower cpm values. With a cut off 450 cpm, the sensitivity of the test is 98%, and the specificity is 97%. The sensitivity increases to 100% with a cutoff of 470 cpm, but specificity decreases to 94%. With the cutoff of 400 cpm, the sensitivity drops to 95%, but the specificity reaches a 100%. Positive predictive accuracy of the test is 95-98%, and the negative predictive accuracy is 99-100%.

Conclusion: Using this method it is possible to detect the difference between the RECAF amounts in cancer sera compared to normal sera with a high degree of specificity and sensitivity (98-100%). This method could find use as a diagnostic tool for blood tests at hospitals for initial cancer detection and also for the follow-up of the patients treated for cancer.

P-12

PROTEASOME INHIBITION HAS A DUAL EFFECT ON HYPOXIC TUMOR CELL RADIOSENSITIVITY

Guy A. Storme, MD, PhD, Mark DeRidder, MD, Dirk L. VandenBerge, MD, Christinne Monsaert, Nathalie Wauters, Valeri N. Verovski, PhD
Cancer Research Unit, Oncologic Center A.Z.-V.U.B., Belgium

Introduction: Transcription factor NF-kB is thought to protect tumor cells from radiation damage by inhibiting apoptosis and by activating DNA repair. Therefore, proteasome inhibition that blocks the early steps of NF-kB activation is considered as a novel strategy to enhance tumor cell radioresponse. However, this approach was developed in aerobic cultures and it remains unclear whether this mechanism is operational in the hypoxic tumor microenvironment. Our recent studies have indicated that the hypoxic tumor cell radiosensitivity may be enhanced through the endogenous generation of NO by inducible nitric oxide synthase (iNOS). Moreover, the iNOS promoter is known to contain specific NF-kB binding sites. We therefore speculated that proteasome inhibition might impair the radiosensitivity of hypoxic tumor cells by down-regulation of iNOS. **Methods:** EMT-6 mammary carcinoma cells were exposed to the proteasome inhibitor lactacystin for 3h and were further incubated with 0.1 µg/ml LPS in 1% oxygen in order to induce iNOS. The hypoxic cell radiosensitivity was estimated by clonogenic assay, the iNOS expression and nuclear NF-kB level by Western blots. The activity of NF-kB was estimated by EMSA using the -984 to -951 base pair radiolabeled consensus of the mouse iNOS promoter and by luciferase reporter gene assay. **Results:** In iNOS positive cells, lactacystin at 20-80 µM caused a concentration-dependent inhibition of nuclear NF-kB expression and activity. Consistently, the expression of iNOS and the hypoxic radiosensitivity were substantially decreased. The impaired radioresponse could be explained by a reduced NO production since the level of nitrite, an oxidative product of NO, was decreased as well. To estimate the radiomodulating effect of proteasome inhibitors in iNOS negative cells, cultures were exposed to lactacystin and further incubated in hypoxia without LPS. Lactacystin caused an evident radiosensitization, but the hypoxic cell radiosensitivity remained considerably lower than that of iNOS positive cells. **Conclusion:** Proteasome inhibitor lactacystin enhances the radioresponse of iNOS negative tumor cells but impairs the radiosensitivity of iNOS positive cells. Since iNOS is expressed in many solid tumors, this mechanism may compromise the radiosensitizing potential of proteasome inhibitors.

P-13

THE NEGATIVE PROGNOSTIC ROLE OF ELEVATED VALUES OF CIRCULATING CROMOGRANIN A (CGA) IN PROSTATE CANCER PATIENTS WITH HORMONE REFRACTORY DISEASE IS NOT LINKED TO A WORSE PSA RESPONSE TO CHEMOTHERAPY

Mirella Torta, MD, Alessandra Mosca, MD, Adriano Priola, MD, Alfredo Berruti, MD, Gabriella Gorzegno, MD, Emiliano Aroasio, MD, Marco Tampellini, MD, Paola Bellati, MD, Cristiano Daglio, MD, Luigi Dogliotti, MD
Oncologia Medica, Dipartimento di Scienze Cliniche e Biologiche, Università degli Studi di Torino; ASO S. Luigi di Orbassano, Laboratorio Analisi, Azienda Ospedaliera San Luigi di Orbassano, Abbott, Divisione Diagnostici, Roma, Italy

The coexistence of neuroendocrine differentiation in prostate cancer patients become refractory to androgen deprivation therapy has been repeatedly correlated with a short survival perspective. The mechanisms of this negative prognostic significance are poorly understood. Neuroendocrine phenotype in prostate cancer population could be easily detected by measuring circulating CgA. Plasma CgA [enzyme-linked immunoadsorbent assay kit; (Dako A/S, Glostrup, Denmark)] and serum prostate specific antigen (PSA), [chemiluminescent method Abbott Architect 2000 (Abbott, Abbott Park, Illinois,USA)] were measured in 48 consecutive prostate cancer patients with hormonal refractory disease before chemotherapy and every 3 months during treatment. Chemotherapy consisted in oral estramustine in 10 patients, estramustine + etoposide in 26 and epirubicin in 12. Elevated CgA (>20 U/L) values at baseline were found in 19 patients (39.6%), 4 of them (8.3%) attained a marker reduction (>50%) during treatment; while 14 (89.6%) obtained a CgA increase. Among the 29 patients with baseline CgA within normality, 19 (65.5%) displayed a marker increase above the threeshold of normality during treatment. More than 50% PSA reduction after chemotherapy was obtained in 14 patients (29.2%). There was a tendency in greater PSA response in patients with elevated CgA (7/19, 36.8%) as opposed to those with normal CgA (7/29, 24.1%) (p=n.s.). Elevated CgA values negatively correlated with overall survival (median 6.1 vs 17.5 months, respectively, p<0.02). To conclude, elevated CgA values in hormone refractory prostate cancer patients are marginally reduced by chemotherapy and significantly correlate with adverse prognosis. The negative prognostic significance of CgA is independent from PSA response.

P-14

UBC II ELISA, AN IMPROVED IMMUNOASSAY FOR MONITORING OF URINARY BLADDER CANCER PATIENTS

Anders Sjodin, BSc, Bo Wiklund, PhD
IDL Biotech AB, Bromma, Sweden

The quantitative UBC II ELISA is a cytokeratin based tumor marker, useful for the management of urinary bladder cancer patients. The measured cytokeratins are epithelial cell specific intermediate filaments that are known to leak from tumor cells during tumorigenesis. By urine analysis of the concentration of cytokeratins 8 and 18, a sensitive measurement of tumor cell activity is obtained for the patient.

A total of 63 urinary bladder cancer patients and 100 apparently healthy individuals were included in the study to evaluate the improved 2nd generation of the UBC test. Spontaneous urine, retained in the bladder for at least 3 hours was collected, centrifuged and stabilized by adding Urine diluent (enclosed) prior to analysis. Apart from sensitivity and specificity of the UBC test, the intra- and interassay precision, and the stability of the kits were analyzed.

The overall sensitivity and specificity for the UBC II test were 79.4% and 95.0%. The 95Th percentile of the apparently healthy individuals was 10.5 µg/l (3.0 ± 6.5 µg/l; median 0.69 µg/l), while the concentration for the urinary bladder cancer patients was 195.1 ± 576.9 µg/l (median 59.2 µg/l). The difference was found to be statistically significant (p<0.001). The positive predictive value (PPV) was 90.9% and the negative predictive value (NPV) 88.0%. Further, biochemical results showed a high intra- and interassay precision for the UBC II test, and in addition a stability of over 12 months was noted.

In conclusion, due to its high sensitivity for urinary bladder cancer, the improved UBC II ELISA tumor marker seems to be of promising additive value in the overall management of urinary bladder cancer patients, where a reduced number of cystoscopies during follow-up of the patients might be possible.

P-15

THE MECHANISMS OF ANTITUMOR IMMUNITY FORMATION DURING XENOTRANSPLANTATION OF TUMOR CELLS INTO AN INERT GEL IMPLANTED SUBCUTANEOUSLY TO MICE

S. E. Severin, A. V. Rodina, E. Yu. Moskaleva, N. V. Gukasova, V. K. Sologub , I. K. Koromyslova, Yu. V. Belousova, I. K. Sviridova, N. S. Sergeeva
Moscow Research Institute of Medical Ecology, Moscow, 113149, Russia Moscow Research Cancer Institute, Moscow, Russia

Our previous studies have demonstrated the possibility of prolonged culturing of xenogeneic tumor cells in rodents with an implanted inert gel. Long-term exposure of mice to alive human tumor cells (human melanoma SK MEL-1) made the mice non-susceptible to syngeneic reinoculated tumors (mouse melanoma B-16). The design of immunotherapeutic methods and/or method of vaccination against human tumors by xenotransplantation (XT) of tumor cells into an inert gel puts forward the necessity to gain a deeper insight into immunological mechanisms underlying the resistance of mice to syngeneic tumors. Therefore, the aim of the present study was to investigate the cytotoxic activity (CTA) of mouse (BDF1) splenocytes in different periods following the injection of human melanoma SK MEL-1 cells into a connective tissue capsule formed around the subcutaneously injected gel by day 60. Histological analysis of the gel surrounded by a vascularized connective tissue capsule revealed the presence of a great number of lymphoid cells. Isolation of these cells and their culturing *in vitro* revealed that these cells contained both lymphocytes and macrophages. The former manifested high CTA activity with respect to B16 cells, whereas 10-40% of macrophages contained melanoma antigens of SK-MEL-1 cells even 3 months after their introduction into the gel. The splenocytes of mice immunized by xenotransplantation of tumor cells (SK MEL-1) into the gel (IXTCG) manifested CTA towards syngeneic tumor cells B16 (STC) from the 3rd day after XT CTA reached the maximum level on day 7 following XT with a subsequent twofold decrease after 2 weeks and remained at this level for at least 12 weeks. High CTA with respect to B16 cells was observed even at low values of the target:effector ratio. Transplantation of tumor cells (B16) to IXTCG and control mice was associated with increased splenocyte CTA levels in early periods (3 days) following reinoculation (the target:effector ratio was 1:2.5 – 1:40). The results obtained testify to a determining role of cell-mediated immunity in the development of antitumor response during immunization with xenogeneic tumor cells transplanted into the connective tissue capsules of mice with subcutaneously implanted inert gel.

P-16

TELOMERE DYSFUNCTION IS INVOLVED IN THE CISPLATIN AND ECTEINASCIDIN-743 SENSITIVITY OF MELANOMA-DERIVED C-MYC LOW-EXPRESSING CLONES

Annamaria Biroccio, PhD, Chiara Gabellini, PhD, Sarah Amodei, PhD, Barbara Benassi, PhD, Donatella Del Bufalo, PhD, Raffaella Elli, PhD, Anna Antonelli, PhD, Maurizio D'Incalci, MD, Gabriella Zupi, PhD
Regina Elena Cancer Institute, Rome, Italy, Cellular Biotechnology and Hematology Department, University "La Sapienza", Rome, Italy, "Istituto di Ricerche Farmacologiche Mario Negri", Milan, Italy

We previously demonstrated that the down-regulation of c-Myc protein expression in M14 melanoma cells increases the susceptibility to cisplatin [cis-diamminedichloroplatinum(II), (CDDP)] and to a novel anticancer drug ecteinascidin-743 (ET-743). Since the decreased c-Myc expression is associated with a concomitant reduction in the human Telomerase Reverse Transcriptase (hTERT) expression and telomerase activity, telomere shortening and dysfunction, the aim of this study was to investigate the role of telomerase function on the ability of c-Myc to modulate the CDDP and ET-743 sensitivity. Reconstitution of hTERT in the c-Myc low-expressing clones restores telomerase activity, reduces telomere dysfunction, and decreases the sensitivity to both drugs. The reduced sensitivity to CDDP and ET-743 is due to the ability of cells to recover from drug-induced damage. Reactivation of telomere function modifies cell cycle progression, enabling the cells to recover from drug-induced G2/M block and consequently protecting them from apoptosis. Taken together these results open the possibility to use c-myc antisense, able to induce telomere dysfunction, followed by telomerase inhibitors and CDDP/ET-743 treatment, to improve the chemotherapeutic response of melanoma.

Supported by grants from Italian Association for Cancer Research (A.I.R.C.), Ministero della Sanità, and CNR-MIUR.

P-17

IMMUNOHISTOCHEMICAL ANALYSIS OF EXPRESSION OF DCC AND NETRIN-1 IN GASTRIC CANCERS

Kimiko Hasegawa, MD, Fumio Itoh, MD, PhD, Yukinari Yoshida, MD, PhD,
Hiroyuki Yamamoto, MD, PhD, Minoru Toyota, MD, PhD, Kohzoh Imai, MD, PhD
Sapporo Medical University, Sapporo, Japan

A body of evidence has been accumulated indicating that reduced or loss of DCC exression is associated with the development of a variety of neoplasms. In this study, we examined DCC expression in 32 gastric cancers by immunohistochemical analysis. At the same time, expression of netrin-1, a ligand of DCC, was immunohistochemically evaluated in normal gastric mucosae and tumor tissues. Overall, reduced expression of DCC was observed in 16 of the tumors (50%). All 5 tumors of poorly differentiated adenocarcinoma of the solid type showed negative staining for DCC. Colocalization of netrin-1 with DCC was mostly observed in normal gastric glands, suggesting that, via DCC, netrin-1 plays some roles in survival or differentiation of gastric epithelial cells, but was because DCC may induce apoptosis in expressing cells that grow or metastasize beyond the limitation of ligand availability.

P-18

LACK OF OLIGONUCLEOSOMAL DNA FRAGMENTATION AND INTRACELLULAR ACIDIFICATION IN IMIDAZOLE-INDUCED APOPTOTIC CELL DEATH

Kazuyuki Hirano, PhD, Kazuhiro Iguchi, Shigeyuki Usui, PhD, Ryoji Ishida, PhD
Gifu Pharmaceutical University, Gifu; Aichi Cancer Center, Nagoya, Japan

Apoptotic process is separated into at least two distinct phases, initiation and execution. The initiation phase involves biochemical changes such as activation of initiator caspases (caspase-8 and 9), mitochondrial dysfunction, and changes in mitochondrial and cytosolic pH, that might be unique to each apoptotic stimulus. These events are well known to contribute to the execution process of apoptosis. On the other hand, the execution phase involves characteristic morphological changes including cell shrinkage, formation of apoptotic bodies, chromatin condensation, and DNA fragmentation. These changes are caused by cleaving multiple intracellular proteins that appear to result from the activation of executioner caspases (caspase-3, 6 and 7). Intracellular acidification is known to be involved in the initiation phase of apoptosis. However, the necessity of intracellular acidic condition in the execution phase of apoptosis remains obscure. To investigate the influence of pHi in the execution phase of apoptosis, we have examined the mode of cell death induced by imidazole, which has been known to affect pHi and apoptotic process. Here, we found that imidazole induces cell death in HL-60 cells, associated with caspase-3 activation and DFF-45 cleavage but not oligonucleosomal DNA fragmentation. We also found that imidazole maintains intracellular pH (pHi) at low level. When pHi was neutralized by changing imidazole-containing medium into fresh medium, oligonucleosomal DNA fragmentation was observed in the imidazole-treated HL-60 cells. Furthermore, this DNA fragmentation induced by intracellular neutralization was inhibited by the treatment with caspase inhibitor. These above results strongly suggest that pHi being maintained in the neutral range is essential for the induction of oligonucleosomal DNA fragmentation in the execution phase of apoptosis.

P-19

QUANTITATIVE ANALYSIS OF SURVIVIN mRNA EXPRESSION IN CANCER SPECIMENS

Daniel M. Kenney, BS, Niranjan Y. Sardesai, PhD, Daniel J. O'Shannessy, PhD
Fujirebio Diagnostics, Inc., Malvern, PA

Survivin is a 16.5 kDa intracellular protein that has been implicated in both inhibition of apoptosis and mitotic regulation. As such considerable recent interest has focused on the potential of survivin as a cancer diagnostic. Indeed survivin over-expression has been demonstrated in a number of tumors, including breast, stomach, pancreas and bladder and appears to plays an important role in cancer progression

We have developed a Taqman(tm) quantitative reverse transcription polymerase chain reaction assay (RT-QPCR) for the measurement of Survivin mRNA. We used endogenous expression levels in a proprietary breast cancer cell line to establish a standard curve and quantify the relative expression levels across samples. Cross-sectional samples consisting of tumor tissues and lymph nodes (n = 18); normal adjacent (to tumor) tissues, normal tissues and peripheral blood leukocytes from apparently healthy donors (n = 14); and cancer cell lines in culture (n = 2) were examined by the RT-QPCR assay.

The assay is both highly specific for tumor presence (14/18 tumors and 13/14 normals correctly identified) and sensitive. Although 123 bp survivin transcripts were detected in all cases, expression levels varied across samples. Survivin mRNA relative expression levels ranged from 0.201 - 1.467 for the tumor samples to 0.006 - 0.089 for normal tissues and PBLs. Thus, the quantitation of Survivin mRNA expression may play an important role in the diagnosis and monitoring of cancer.

P-20

A NEW ARCHIVABLE SUBNANO SCALE NUCLEIC ACID AMPLIFICATION METHOD FOR GENE EXPRESSION PROFILING

Simon W. Law, Haisun Liao, Natalia Mamaeva, Amy Deik, Tai-nang Huang
Linden Technologies, Inc., Woburn, MA

DNA Microarray has rapidly become an essential tool for high throughput gene expression and other genomic studies. Investigators can now study thousands of genes in one experiment. This led to many powerful and exciting advances in our understanding of human diseases, by providing a signature of the genetic expression profile of the disease tissue. Global expression studies such as gene expression profiling are possible when the investigators have access to enough samples to do the experiments. A typical glass slide cDNA or oligoarray analysis requires 30-50 ug total RNA per slide. Disease tissues are usually heterogeneous, and sample complexity sets a limit as to what kind of questions might be addressed. Recently, a few linear amplification methods, which are modifications of the original Eberwine T7 RNA polymerase transcription procedure has been developed to address the small sample issues. However, all these methods are solution based, therefore, the original sample can only be used once. Furthermore, the amplification power of currently available methods can produce barely enough material from a few hundred cells, such as those derived from laser captured microdissection (LCM) samples. We hypothesized that solid phase amplification should allow for archiving of the original sample, and that it may be just as robust as solution-based methods. To assess feasibility, we designed two anchor primers and a universal tag sequence. The anchor primer serve as capture as well as amplification cassette. The universal tag sequence provides an affinity tag for anchor primer capture. Starting with 1 ng of total RNA, we obtained $3x10e^8$ fold amplification. The bound nucleic acid can be amplified repeatedly over a period of at least 4 months with no observable skewing of expression profile, demonstrating archivability. The method is easy to perform and automatable. We believe this technology, which we called SPTCR, will be very useful in genetic analysis. Details of the technology will be discussed.

P-21

METHYLATION ANALYSIS OF THE CPG ISLANDS IN THE PROMOTER REGIONS OF THE CDX1, CDX2 AND SOX-2 GENES IN INTESTINAL METAPLASIA OF THE HUMAN STOMACH

Mami Mihara, MD, Ken-ichi Inada, MD, PhD, Tetsuya Tsukamoto, MD, PhD, Kohzoh Imai, MD, PhD, Takashi Sugimura, MD, PhD, Masae Tatematsu, MD, PhD, Toshikazu Ushijima, MD, PhD
Carcinogenesis Division, National Cancer Center Res. Institute, Tokyo; Division of Oncology Pathology, Aichi Cancer Center Res. Institute, Nagoya; 1st Department Internal Medicine, Sapporo Medical University, Sapporo, Japan

Intestinal metaplasia (IM) of the stomach is known as aberrant differentiation of gastric epithelium into intestinal epithelium. It is known that two intestine-specific homeobox genes, Cdx1, Cdx2, are aberrantly expressed in IM, and we have recently found that expression of a stomach-specific homeobox gene, SOX-2, is decreased in IM. Here, involvements of the changes in CpG methylations, which are considered to be involved in tissue differentiation, were analyzed. Pyloric glands with IM and those without IM were isolated by the gland isolation technique, and methylation statuses were analyzed by methylation-specific PCR (MSP). The CpG islands (CGIs) in the promoter regions of Cdx1 and Cdx2 were demethylated regardless of the presence or absence of IM. On the other hand, the CGI in the promoter region of SOX-2 was found to be methylated in the pyloric glands with IM while it was demethylated in the pyloric glands without IM. The role of the SOX-2 methylation in its decreased expression is being investigated. These finding suggested that aberrant methylation of a key gene(s) in tissue differentiation could be involved in aberrant tissue differentiation like IM.

P-22

PAN-TUMORAL RECOGNITION BY AN AFP RECEPTOR ASSAY KIT

E.B. Song, G. Shen, X. Hu, A. Kummer, C. Chen and R. Moro
Pacific Biosciences Research Centre, Vancouver, Canada

The AFP receptor (RECAF) mediates the binding and uptake of AFP by a variety of fetal and cancer cells, but not by normal adult cells. This behavior defines RECAF as a widespread oncofetal antigen. Our group has developed, under contract with BioCurex Inc. (Rancho Santa Margarita, CA), a commercial kit (the BioCurex Histo-RECAF™ kit) for the detection of cancer cells on tissue sections. Using this single step kit, we stained paraffin embedded samples of breast, lung, stomach and prostate cancers. In all cases, we found a clear difference between the staining of cancer cells as compared to non-malignant cells in all tissue preparations. The staining was granular and always cytoplasmic and in some cases, it was accompanied by capping on the cell membrane and the nuclear membrane, suggesting that the AFP receptor system might be involved in the transmission of signals from the extracellular environment to the cell nucleus. The staining intensity varied from one cluster of cancer cells to another, as well as among the individual cells within a given cluster in various tissue preparations. Morphologically normal or displastic cells were, in their immense majority, completely negative. Lymphoid structures within specimens were negative, unless cancer cells invaded them. In a stomach cancer case, a staining gradient was observed from the normal glands, which were completely negative to the carcinoma cells, which were strongly positive. Adjusting the reagent concentrations, we were able to produce a version of this kit that only requires a 5-10 minute incubation for use on intra-operative frozen sections.

P-23

OVEREXPRESSION OF ALPHA-FETOPROTEIN IN HEPG2 CELLS

C.S. Russell, C. Chen and R. Moro
Pacific Biosciences Research Centre, Vancouver, Canada

A common source of human alpha-fetoprotein (AFP) is the human hepatoma cell line HepG2. To increase AFP production, we introduced engineered DNA constructs in that cell line. Unigene was used to identify DNA clones that appeared to have identity with the 2.2 kilobase human AFP cDNA sequence (Genebank V01514). A suitable clone was introduced into a mammalian cDNA expression vector, which includes a neomycin resistance cassette allowing for selection of clones with integrated transgene constructs. A G418 death curve was established for HepG2 and 1 mg/ml was determined to kill non-transfected cells in 8 days. Cells were transfected with the AFP DNA construct, G418 selection was introduced 24 hours later and maintained for 20 days until individual cell clones were evident to the naked eye. Individual clones were picked and amplified with continual G418 selection. Serum free medium was used to increase AFP synthesis relative to albumin and to facilitate AFP isolation. AFP protein expression was quantified and normalized to cell viability.

Results: Expression of human AFP was increased to ~130 mg/ml (~400% increase) in the culture medium. The rate of AFP production was also increased relative to non-transfected cells. High level AFP expression appeared to be stable especially in the presence of G418 selection. The recombinant AFP is antigenically similar or identical to non-transfected HepG2 derived AFP as shown by an AFP commercial kit.

P-24

MILK COMPONENT COMPETES WITH AFP FOR RECEPTOR SITE

Natashia Webb, Ricardo Moro
Pacific Biosciences Research Center, Richmond, British Columbia, Canada

Alpha-fetoprotein (AFP) is produced in the liver and it circulates in high concentrations during human development. It has been shown that AFP is incorporated into fetal and malignant cells via a receptor (RECAF). AFP also binds to malignant cell extracts as evidenced in a simple binding assay in which 96 well microtiter plates are coated with cell extract, blocked with a blocking agent, and detected by adding labeled AFP.

When 5% milk is utilized as the blocking agent, binding of AFP to its receptor site is almost completely lost. Further investigation revealed that serial milk dilutions produce an inhibition curve in the range of 0.1-0.001%. The same effect is observed on plates coated with RECAF purified on an AFP affinity column. Various extracts from cancer cell lines including MCF-7 (breast), K562 (leukemia), H292 (lung), and CaoV3 (ovarian) yield similar results. Fresh and reconstituted skim milk, as well as human milk samples were tested to determine if the observed phenomenon was common among various sources and processing procedures. All milk samples exhibited the same behavior, however human milk to a lesser degree. The molecule interacting with the receptor is larger then 6-8kDa since dialysis did not eliminate the effect. Whey produced by treatment of milk with acetic acid to remove the casein micelles followed by boiling for 30 minutes displayed identical behavior. Precipitation of whey proteins using 20% trichloroacetic acid had no effect on the inhibitory molecule, however digestion of whey with 0.2% pepsin resulted in total loss of the inhibitory effect.

These results provide evidence for the existence of a naturally occurring molecule in bovine and human milk that competes with AFP for binding to its receptor RECAF.

P-25

MODIFIED FORMS OF THE EGF RECEPTOR-BINDING FRAGMENT AS AN EFFICIENT VEHICLE FOR TARGETED DRUG DELIVERY TO TUMOR CELLS

S. V. Lutsenko, S. M. Kiselev, N. B. Feldman, D. V. Zabolotnev, S. E. Severin
Moscow Research Institute of Medical Ecology, Moscow, Russia

The receptor-binding fragment of the epidermal growth factor, $EGFfr_{20\text{-}31}$, and its two modified forms, EGFfr 1 and EGFfr 2, have been synthesized. EGFfr 1 differed from the original fragment by the presence of Ser instead of Lys in position 28. EGFfr 2 contained Lys instead of Met in position 20 and Ser instead of Lys in position 28. Both modified fragments manifested biological activities during stimulation of proliferation of NIH3T3 fibroblasts *in vitro* which were close to that of $EGFfr_{20\text{-}31}$. To ensure targeted delivery of doxorubicin (DR) to tumor cells, DR conjugates with $EGFfr_{20\text{-}31}$, EGFfr 1 and EGFfr 2 were synthesized with the help of the bifunctional crosslinking reagent SPDP. The peptide:DR molar ratio of each conjugate was 1:1. All the conjugates manifested cytotoxic activities towards cultured tumor cells (HeLa) *in vitro* which exceeded that of the free antibiotic 2–4-fold. This suggests that the amino acid substitutions in the $EGFfr_{20\text{-}31}$ fragment are responsible for the loss of its receptor-binding ability. All the conjugates under study can be used for targeted delivery of DR and, perhaps, some other antitumor drugs, to tumor cells.

P-26

TUMOR GROWTH SUPPRESSION BY APOPTOSIS INDUCED WITH ANTI-ERBB-2 CHIMERIC MONOCLONAL ANTIBODY

Masayuki Tsujisaki, MD, PhD, Sigeru Sasaki, MD, PhD, Hiromi Hirata, MD, PhD,
Yasuo Katoh, MD, PhD, Toshio Matsune, PhD, Kohzoh Imai, MD, PhD
First Department of Internal Medicine, Sapporo Medical University, Shirakaba Pharmacy
Sapporo, Japan

ErbB-2, a member of the epidermal growth factor(EGF) receptor tyrosine kinase family,is often overexpressed and/or amplified in breast,ovarian and gastric cancers and other malignancies. ErbB-2 is a candidate as one of the best target molecules for cancer therapy. We established an anti-erbB-2 mouse-human chimeric monoclonal antibody(MoAb) CH401,which was able to kill cancer cells overexpressing the erbB-2 protein in vitro. The analysis of the killing mechanism indicated that MoAb CH401 might be the first anti-erbB-2 mouse-human chimeric MoAb which can induce the apoptosis of cancer cells, since morphological changes and DNA fragmentation were recognized in MoAb CH401-treatedcells. The study in vivo showed that erbB-2 transfected SV22 cells did not form tumors at all in SCID mice treated with MoAb CH401 alone. Apoptosis signaling in erbB-2 positive cells induced by MoAb CH401 were investigated;CH401 activates the JNK and p38 MAPKinase pathway,and down-regulates ERK pathway. These results may suggest that MoAb CH401 has a therapeutic potential for erbB-2 overexpressing cancers. This approach may be particularly valuable as a new type of cancer therapy.

P-27

ENDOTHELIAL CELL GROWTH SUPPRESSING FACTOR EXHIBITS TUMOR REGRESSING ACTIVITY

Shigeyuki Usui, PhD, Kazuyuki Hirano, PhD
Department of Pharmaceutics, Gifu Pharmaceutical University, Gifu, Japan

A carboxymethylated derivertive of a linear (1-3)-b-D-glucan (CMCD) from Alcaligenes faecalis var. myxogenes acted directly on mouse peritoneal macrophages and mouse lymphoma P388D1 cells, and induced a growth suppressing activity for bovine artery endothelial cells (BAE) from themselves. An endothelial cell growth-suppressing factor (EGSF) was purified from the conditioned medium of a P388D1 cell culture in the presence of CMCD. The purification steps included, in order, ammonium sulfate fractionation and six stages of column chromatography on Macro-Prep Ceramic Hydroxyapatite, Q-Sepharose, Sephacryl S-300 HR, Matrex PBA-30, PBE94, and, anti-bovine serum albumin agarose. The purified EGSF showed two bands with silver staining on a SDS-polyacrylamide gel under reducing conditions and their molecular masses were estimated as approximately 55 and 63 kDa, while the molecular mass of the purified EGSF was estimated as about 65 kDa by gel filtration using Superdex 200HR. This factor strongly suppressed the proliferation of endothelial cells from bovine artery, human umbilical vein, and human dermal vas capillare and this suppression was observed to be reversible. The intravenous administration of the purified EGSF to sarcoma 180-bearing mouse caused a rapid decrease in the number of viable tumor cells in tumor lumps within 16 h and immunohistochemical study demonstrated that hemorrhagic disorder all over the tissue in the tumor lamp occurred. Thus, the purified factor exhibited not only growth suppressing activity for endothelial cells but also tumor regressing activity. The purified factor significantly inhibited in vitro tubulogenesis of bovine artery, human umbilical vein, and adult human dermal microvascular endothelial cells on collagen gel. After the tube formation of endothelial cells was completed on a collagen gel, the purified factor disrupted the tubes. These findings demonstrate that EGSF is a potent inhibitor of angiogenesis as well as the growth of endothelial cells, and may bring about the regression of a solid tumor by inhibiting angiogenesis.

P-28

SERRATED ADENOMA PHENOTYPE AND K-RAS CODON 12 MUTATION IN COLORECTAL ADENOMAS

Shi Yang, MD, Elizabeth Mulcahy, MD, Conor O'Keane, MD, Michael J O'Brien, MPH
Boston University School of Medicine, Boston, MA

Background: Serrated adenoma is an adenoma variant that is thought to evolve from a precursor hyperplastic polyp. K-ras mutations are frequent in villous adenomas and in distally located hyperplastic polyps. In this study we compared the frequency of k-ras mutation in adenomas with and without a serrated phenotype.

Method: A series of 64 endoscopically and surgically resected adenomas were classified as tubular, tubulovillous and villous adenomas according to the extent of the villous component,and by size, presence of high grade dysplasia and location. They were further categorized as showing serrated phenotype if any of the following features were present: 1. Surface absorptive cell differentiation of villi. 2. Non-branching villi or 3. Villi with a serrated outline. A PCR-R++FLP method was used to identify the k-ras codon 12 mutation from adenoma DNA extracted from paraffin sections. MIB1 staining was performed to evaluate proliferative activity.

Result: The mean size of the adenomas was 2.0 centimeter. Mean proliferation index was 32.1%. K-ras mutation was strongly associated with adenomas larger than 2.0-centimeters ($p=0.005$, OR=6.2) and villous growth pattern ($p=0.004$, OR=5.3). The strongest association among the factors evaluated was found between k-ras mutation and serrated phenotype ($p<0.0001$, OR = 25.3). Eighty percent(80%) of adenomas with k-ras mutations showed serrated phenotype as compared to 13.6 % of adenomas that lacked such features.

Conclusion: Serrated phenotype is strongly associated with k-ras mutation in colorectal adenomas. Our findings suggest the hypothesis that a proportion of villous adenomas may evolve from k-ras positive hyperplastic polyps or serrated adenomas

P-29

ANTITUMOR EFFECT OF RESVERATROL ON HUMAN MELANOMA CELL LINES

Maria Pia Fuggetta, PhD, Giulia Lanzilli, PhD, Maria Tricarico, PhD, Stefania D'Atri, PhD, Elena Cannavo, PhD, Roberto Falchetti, PhD
Institute of Neurobiology and Molecular Medicine. CNR; Istituto Dermopatico Immacolata IRCCS, Rome, Italy

Background: Resveratrol, a natural polyphenolic phytoalexine, found in grapes and other plants has been reported to be a potent antioxidant, anti-platelet, anti-inflammatory and antiproliferative agent that is thought to have chemopreventive properties. The aim of the present study was to evaluate the in vitro effects of trans-resveratrol (T-Res, trans-3,4',5-trihydroxystilbene) on human melanoma.

Methods: T-Res was tested in vitro on four melanoma cell lines: M14, SKMEL-28, PR-Mel, GR-Mel in a dose range of 5-40 mcg/ml. The effects of this compound were evaluated at different times of culture on: 1) tumor cell growth, 2) cell cycle kinetics, 3) pro-apoptotic activity.

Results: 1)Data obtained by MTT and trypan blue dye exclusion methods show that T-Res induces a significant antiproliferative effect in a time- and dose- dependent manner on all lines examined although a differential susceptibility among the four melanoma tested was observed. In any case, when compared with the in vitro treatment with BCNU or Temozolomide, the conventional drug for melanoma therapy, the inhibitory effect of T-Res appears to be more efficient in inhibiting tumor growth. 2)T-Res treatment of melanoma cells results in a significant dose-related accumulation in the S phase of cell cycle. 3)In the same culture conditions the treatment with T-Res induces apoptosis as demonstrated by flow cytometry and PARP cleavage. Taken together these findings suggest that T-Res has a strong potential for its development as an agent for therapy and prevention of melanoma. (Supported by Provincia Autonoma di Trento,Italy)

P-30

ALPHA-FETOPROTEIN POSITIVELY REGULATES THE CYTOCHROME C-MEDIATED FORMATION OF THE APAF-1 APOPTOSOME COMPLEX IN A CELL-FREE SYSTEM

Lidia N. Semenkova, PhD, Elena I. Dudich, PhD, Igor V. Dudich, PhD, Natalie A. Tokhtamisheva, PhD, Timo K. Korpela, PhD
Institute of Immunological Engineering, Lyubuchany, Russia

Mitochondrial apoptosis pathway is mediated via cytochrome c release with subsequent formation of the Apaf-1/cyt-c/dATP/procaspase-9 complex, leading to activation of caspase-9 and downstream effector caspase-3. Our recent data demonstrated that oncoembrionic marker alpha-fetoprotein (AFP) could synergistically enhance caspase-9 and caspase-3 activation in cell-free cytosolic extracts of tumor cells in the presence of the sub-optimal dose of endogenous or exogenous cyt-c. We therefore proposed that AFP might physically associate with the apoptosome and enhance caspase-3 activation in the complex. High-resolution gel chromatography of the cyt-c/dATP-activated cell-free cytosolic extract of HepG2 cells demonstrated that addition of AFP was resulted in the notable changes in the distribution of the caspase-3 activity along the gel-filtration elution pattern. Thus, it was observed that AFP induced significant enhance of the caspase-3 activity in the region of the biologically active Mr ~ 700 kDa apoptosome complex and stimulated release of the active caspase-3 from the complex. Distribution of the activity of caspase-9 was not affected by AFP treatment. By immunoblotting we have detected active degradation of the Apaf-1 yielded the small ~35 kDa C-terminal fragment in the course of cyt-c-mediated formation of the active Mr ~ 700 kDa apoptosome complex. Addition of AFP together with low doses of cyt-c/dATP resulted in the significant decrease of the amount of the fragmented Apaf-1 in the region of Mr ~ 700 kDa apoptosome complex. Simultaneously, it was observed that AFP affects distribution of the inhibitor-of-apoptosis-proteins along the chromatography pattern of the apoptosome assembly to displace IAP-2 from the 700-kDa apoptosome comlex. It is concluded that AFP positively regulates apoptosome formation, caspase-3 activation and preserves Apaf-1 from caspase-dependent degradation. The precise mechanism by which AFP enhances caspase-3 activity remains to be elucidated. It is suggested that AFP might operate by abrogation of action of IAPs.

P-31

STRUCTURAL REQUIREMENTS FOR TRIGGERING OF AFP-MEDIATED APOPTOSIS IN TUMOR CELLS. MODULATION OF FUNCTIONAL ACTIVITY OF AFP BY CONFORMATIONAL CHANGES

Igor V. Dudich, PhD, Elena I. Dudich, PhD, Lidia N. Semenkova, PhD, Natalie A. Tokhtamisheva, PhD,
Ykka Hellmann, PhD,Timo K.Korpela, PhD
Institute of Immunological Engineering, Lyubuchany, Russia

Comparative study of the general protein structure and functional activity of the human a-fetoprotein (AFP), ligand-free AFP and AFP loaded with arachidonic acid (AA) or estradiol (E2) was carried out. By circular dichroism it was shown that secondary structure of the AFP molecule did not depend on the presence of noncovalently-bound ligands. By differential scanning calorimetry it was demonstrated that thermodynamic parameters of the AFP molecule, such as denaturation enthalpy and temperature of the denaturation transition, which are the characteristics of the molecular tertiary structure, critically depend on the presence of AFP-bound ligands and concentration-dependent equilibrium protein dimerization, showing the reversible conformational change in the AFP tertiary structure induced by ligand removal or homodimerization. It was also demonstrated that thermal denaturation of AFP molecule includes two independent highly cooperative transitions suggesting a two-domain structure for intact AFP macromolecule. Comparative studies of the various conformational forms of the AFP and its peptic fragments for their ability to induce apoptosis of cancer cells demonstrated distinct correlation between tertiary structure and functional activity. It was shown that: (i) concentration-dependent AFP homodimerisation that is occurs via formation of heterodimeric complex of C- and N-terminal domains is necessary to form the functional active site responsible for apoptosis induction; (ii) AFP-mediated cell growth regulation is an activity intrinsic to the molecule itself and cannot be attributed to either putative non-covalently bound ligands; (iii) biologically active ligand molecules may however positively, or negatively modulate AFP-mediated cell growth regulative activity.